FIFTH EDITION

CARE PLANNING POCKET GUIDE

A NURSING DIAGNOSIS APPROACH

JANET REISS LEDERER, MN, RN
Manager, Patient and Community Health Education
El Camino Hospital, Mountain View, California

GAIL L. MARCULESCU, MS, RN, CETN
Enterostomal Therapy Nurse Coordinator
El Camino Hospital, Mountain View, California

BARBARA MOCNIK, MS, RN
Program Manager, Psychiatry/Behavioral Medicine Services
El Camino Hospital, Mountain View, California

NANCY SEABY, MS, RN
Staff Development and Quality Assurance Specialist,
Dialysis Services
El Camino Hospital, Mountain View, California

ADDISON-WESLEY NURSING
A Division of The Benjamin/Cummings Publishing Company, Inc.
Redwood City, California • Menlo Park, California • Reading, Massachusetts
New York • Don Mills, Ontario • Wokingham, U.K. • Amsterdam • Bonn
Sydney • Singapore • Tokyo • Madrid • San Juan

Executive Editor: Patti Cleary
Project Editor: Bradley Burch
Senior Production Supervisor: Judith Hibbard
Cover Designer: John Martucci
Text Designer: Eleanor Mennick
Copyeditor: Wendy Earl
Proofreader: David W. Rich
Indexer: Elinor Lindheimer
Compositor: The Cowans

Care has been taken to confirm the accuracy of information presented in this book. The authors, editors, and publisher, however, cannot accept any responsibility for errors or omissions or for consequences from application of the information in this book and make no warranty, express or implied, with respect to its contents.

Library of Congress Cataloging-in-Publication Data
Care planning pocket guide : a nursing diagnosis approach /
  Janet Reiss Lederer . . . [et al.].— 5th ed.
      p.   cm.
   Includes bibliographical references and index.
   ISBN 0-8053-4104-8
1. Nursing care plans—Handbooks, manuals, etc.   2. Nursing
diagnosis—Handbooks, manuals, etc.   I. Lederer, Janet Reiss, 1944–   .
   [DNLM: 1. Nursing Diagnosis—handbooks.   2. Patient Care
Planning—handbooks.   WY 39 C271]
RT49.C37   1993
610.73—dc20
DNLM/DLC
for Library of Congress   92-48222
                                                              CIP

1 2 3 4 5 6 7 8 9 10 MU 97 96 95 94 93

Addison-Wesley Nursing
A Division of The Benjamin/Cummings Publishing Company, Inc.
390 Bridge Parkway
Redwood City, California 94065

■ Contents

■ Preface

The *Care Planning Pocket Guide* is an educational tool and practical guide designed to help nurses develop individualized nursing care plans. In this fifth edition, the general format remains the same as that of the first edition of the book. The content, however, has been expanded to include all nursing diagnoses approved by the North American Nursing Diagnosis Association through May, 1992. The content includes medical, surgical, psychiatric, perinatal, and pediatric patient populations. A variety of special features contributes to the book's usefulness and makes it an indispensable tool for writing care plans.

Features

Organized for easy use   The book is divided into two main parts: (1) Complete plans of care, written according to nursing diagnoses; and (2) a list of medical, surgical, psychiatric, perinatal, and pediatric conditions, each accompanied by suggested nursing diagnoses. This unique organization allows the nurse to begin the care planning process with either a medical condition or a nursing diagnosis.

Suggested alternative diagnoses   Most care plans list suggested alternative diagnoses that the nurse may review to select the most appropriate patient-specific nursing diagnosis.

Easy to individualize   Each nursing diagnosis has suggested "related factors" or "risk factors" that make it easy to individualize the care plan to the specific patient situation. The authors encourage creativity by suggesting that nurses add specific outcomes, interventions, and "related factors" or "risk factors" in order to tailor the care plan to the individual patient.

Comprehensive   Each plan of care is comprehensive and allows nurses to select specific content according to the patient's condition and situation. Each plan includes (1) the "related factors" or "risk factors," (2) a definition of the nursing diagnosis, (3) defining characteristics, (4) suggested alternative diagnoses, (5) expected outcomes, (6) a reminder to specify the frequency of documentation and expected date of completion, and (7) suggested nursing interventions.

Audience   This handbook was developed to facilitate care planning for nursing students, staff nurses in a variety of settings, clinical nurse specialists, and staff development instructors.

The novice care planner, or the experienced nurse less familiar with nursing diagnosis, may find it helpful to begin with the list of medical, surgical, psychiatric, perinatal, and pediatric conditions. Once the nursing diagnoses have been selected, the nurse can use the plans of care to formulate individualized, patient-centered care plans. The nurse who is more familiar with the care planning process will find the content in both sections useful in formulating new and creative care plans. The expert in nursing care planning will be able to use this book to extract information that further expresses the needs of the patient and/or family in a variety of settings.

■ Introduction

Background

In 1973, nursing diagnosis was formalized when the American Nurses Association mandated the use of nursing diagnosis in nursing practice. Invited clinicians, educators, researchers, and theorists from every area of nursing practice came together to offer labels for conditions they had observed in practice. From this beginning, the North American Nursing Diagnosis Association (NANDA) was established as the formal body for the promotion, review, and endorsement of the current list of nursing diagnoses used by practicing nurses. The NANDA membership convenes every two years to consider revisions and additions to the list of nursing diagnoses. The current list of about 110 diagnoses will undoubtedly expand as nurses explore the breadth and depth of nursing practice.

As the list of nursing diagnoses expanded, NANDA developed a classification system, Taxonomy I, which "groups the diagnoses into classes and subclasses so that patterns and relationships among them can emerge" (1992, Taxonomy I, Revised, p. 1). As Taxonomy I has been revised and expanded, NANDA, working in conjunction with the American Nurses' Association, proposed that the Taxonomy be included in the World Health Organization International Classification of Diseases (ICD), Tenth Revision. This proposal was not approved for ICD–10; however, work continues to incorporate nursing diagnosis in ICD revisions. Inclusion of Taxonomy I in the ICD would represent a milestone for nursing by recognizing the significant conditions that require nursing care, more clearly defining nursing's scope of practice, and providing a mechanism for reimbursement of nursing care.

The Value of Nursing Diagnosis

Nursing diagnosis benefits the nursing profession because it helps define the scope of nursing practice by describing conditions the nurse can independently and legally treat. Nursing diagnosis highlights critical thinking and decision-making in the nursing process.

The importance of nursing diagnosis is supported by nurses both in professional literature and in clinical practice. Nursing diagnosis provides a consistent and universally understood terminology among nurses working in various settings, including hospitals, the community, extended care facilities, occupational health facilities, and private practice.

Nursing Process in Relation to Nursing Diagnosis

Using the nursing process to create a plan of care provides a structure for nursing practice and is, in fact, the essence of nursing. The nursing process is put to use continuously during the rendering of nursing care in every clinical setting. Many components of the nursing process overlap and often are repeated, making all aspects of nursing care dynamic. It is important to consider the patient as the central figure in the plan of care. The nurse must confirm the appropriateness of all aspects of nursing care by observing the patient's response to the interventions, be they medical, surgical, or psychosocial.

What process is used to determine the appropriate diagnostic statement for the patient? Data collection and assessment are imperative as the initial steps in the critical thinking and decision making that may lead to the identification of a nursing diagnosis. The definition and defining characteristics of the nursing diagnosis assist the nurse in validating the diagnosis. Once the nursing diagnosis and the "related factors" or "risk factors" are determined, the plan of care is created. The nurse selects the relevant patient outcome statement, including the patient's perceptions and suggestions for the outcome, if possible. Only those patient outcomes that are specific to the patient are selected; not all outcomes apply to every situation. After identifying the outcomes, the nurse includes the patient, whenever possible, to determine which interventions will help the patient achieve the stated outcomes. It is necessary to choose only those interventions that address the etiology of the problem and help return the patient to optimal health.

Evaluation is a component of each step of the nursing process. Is the nursing diagnosis still appropriate? Has the patient achieved the desired outcome? Are the documentation interval and the target date still appropriate and realistic? Are certain interventions no longer needed? The nurse needs to ask these questions to determine whether changes are needed in the individualized plan of care.

Standards of Care in Relation to Nursing Diagnosis

There is an interrelationship between nursing diagnosis care planning and standards of care. Standards of care are developed for a group of patients about whom generalized predictions can be made. These standards direct a set of common nursing interventions for specific patient groups. Where there are written standards of care, nursing diagnosis care planning is not used to communicate routine nursing interventions. Nursing diagnosis care planning is used for those exceptional patient problems that are not addressed in the standards of care.

Managed Care and Case Management in Relation to Nursing Diagnosis

Escalating health care costs and the demand for health care reform have provoked a restructuring of traditional care delivery systems and practice patterns. Two multidisciplinary clinical systems (reform strategies implemented in some health care settings since the mid-1980s) are Managed Care and Case Management. Objectives of a restructured care delivery system may include:

1. To achieve the following high-quality patient outcomes within an appropriate timeframe:
   - Patient wellness
   - Patient/family self-care skills
   - Patient/family satisfaction
2. To establish collaborative practice and improve service coordination and continuity of care
3. To use health care resources appropriately
4. To direct the contributions of all care providers toward the achievement of patient outcomes
5. To increase job satisfaction and job enrichment for caregivers
6. To encourage innovation and ongoing integration of advances in health care

In Managed Care delivery systems, a new tool called a "critical path" has been developed to facilitate achievement of anticipated patient and family outcomes. The critical path is an outline of crucial multidisciplinary activities performed by nurses, physicians, and other members of the health care team that occurs within a predictable and established timeframe. When the expected outcomes are not achieved within the anticipated timeframe, a "variance" occurs and requires analysis. Variances may arise from a variety of sources, including the system (both internal and external to the institution), the practitioner, and/or the patient.

In Managed Care, critical paths standardize practice for the common, usual, and most prevalent case types. In addition, Managed Care provides the foundation for Case Management, a system that uses health care professionals to coordinate care for high-risk, complex populations who may use a disproportionate share of health care resources. The Case Manager focuses on roles and relationships and provides a well coordinated care experience for patients and families in all settings in which the patient receives care.

In Managed Care and Case Management systems, patient care is planned using the multidisciplinary critical path rather than the traditional nursing care plan. In the absence of a traditional nursing care plan, some delivery systems have incorporated nursing diagnosis directly into the critical path, whereas others have used nursing diagnosis to name variance and develop an individualized plan for achieving revised outcomes. For example, incorporating nursing diagnosis into a critical path for the newly diagnosed insulin-dependent diabetic may include the nursing diagnosis

Knowledge Deficit:
related to limited exposure to information and limited practice of skill as evidenced by verbalization of limited knowledge, inaccurate follow-through of instruction, and inaccurate performance on tests.

The expected outcomes may be that by day 3, the patient will recognize signs and symptoms of hypo/hyperglycemia, and by day 5, be prepared to self-inject the required dose of insulin.

When nursing diagnosis is used to name variance, a critical path for this patient would not include a nursing diagnosis, but rather would list "teaching needs" for each day. On day 5, if the patient is unable to meet the outcome of self-injection, this variance is identified and analyzed. A nursing diagnosis such as *Ineffective Individual Coping* might be used to individualize the nursing care for this patient's variance from the critical path.

In organizations with Managed Care and/or Case Management, the customary vehicle for nursing diagnosis—the traditional nursing care plan—does not exist. However, the authors believe that nursing diagnosis will find its appropriate place in multidisciplinary care planning. It is vital that today's nurse be well versed in the use of nursing diagnosis in order to work with the multidisciplinary team to effectively identify and address nursing care issues in restructured care delivery systems.

■ Components of Nursing Diagnosis Care Plans

This book is organized into two parts: "Plans of Care" and "Clinical Conditions Guide to Nursing Diagnoses." More specific information regarding these two parts, with some examples of how to use them, follows.

Plans of Care

Each plan of care includes a nursing diagnostic statement (with its definition), defining characteristics, suggested alternative diagnoses, "related factors" or "risk factors," measurable patient outcomes, documentation intervals and target dates, and nursing interventions.

NANDA organizes nursing diagnoses according to a conceptual framework found in Taxonomy I Revised (see Appendix). Since the goal of this text is to provide a ready reference for the practicing nurse, the nursing diagnosis care plans are organized alphabetically instead of by the taxonomy. Some of the titles were reworded as well, to set forth the key concept in the first word of the title. For example, *Individual Coping, Ineffective* is more easily found in an index when it is written *Coping, Ineffective Individual.*

All approved NANDA (May 1992) diagnoses are included as separate care plans. However, the authors have chosen to modify the standard care plan format for select diagnoses, believing that these particular diagnostic categories are too broad for one care plan. For diagnoses listed below, therefore, care plans in this text include the related factors or risk factors, definition, and defining characteristics. From there, the nurse is referred to other care plans for patient outcomes and interventions.

Disuse Syndrome: High Risk

Tissue Integrity, Impaired

Tissue Perfusion, Altered: Renal, Cerebral, Cardiopulmonary, Gastrointestinal

Thermoregulation, Impaired

Urinary Elimination, Altered

The authors did not separate the nursing diagnosis *Self-Care Deficit: Bathing/ Hygiene, Dressing/Grooming, Feeding,Toileting* into distinct care plans because the format, as it stands, provides the opportunity to specify the self-care deficit and to select concomitant outcomes and interventions.

Components of the care plan are described under the following headings:

Nursing diagnosis

The nursing diagnosis is a concise phrase or label that describes patient conditions observed in practice. These conditions may be actual or potential problems. NANDA has identified seventeen potential problems that in this text are labeled *High Risk.*

Related factors

The related factors imply a link or connection to the nursing diagnosis. Such factors may be described as "related to," "antecedent to," "associated with," "contributing to," or "abetting." The factors delineate what should change for the patient to return to optimal health. Accurately identifying the related factor assists the nurse in selecting interventions appropriate to the desired outcome. As an example, for the diagnosis *Activity Intolerance,* the nursing interventions for a patient whose related factor is arrhythmias would be very different from the interventions for a patient whose related factor is chronic pain.

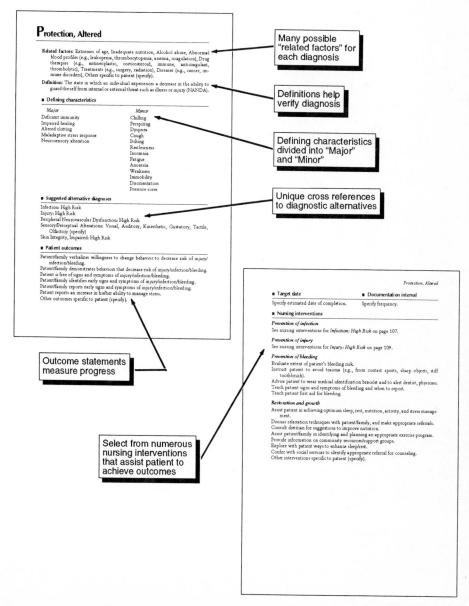

Risk factors

Risk factors will be found only in the high-risk nursing diagnoses. Unlike the related factors described above, a cluster of risk factors contributes to the patient's potential problem, only some of which may be influenced by nursing care. The risk factors are similar to related factors and defining characteristics in the development of the care plan. They describe events and behaviors that put the patient at risk and suggest interventions to protect the patient. As an example, an elderly patient might be diagnosed with *Trauma: High Risk* who exhibits the following risk factors: weakness, poor vision, balancing difficulties, slippery floors, and unanchored rugs. This cluster of risk factors suggests the need for interventions to prevent falls.

Definition

The definition of each nursing diagnosis helps the nurse verify a particular nursing diagnosis. Most definitions were developed by NANDA (Taxonomy I Revised); others were adapted by the authors from NANDA and other sources, and a few are the original definitions of the authors. The source is cited after each definition. Those definitions where no source is cited are the original work of the authors.

Defining characteristics

Defining characteristics are descriptors of patient behavior, either observed by the nurse or verbalized by the patient/family. Frequently discovered during the initial nursing history and assessment, the defining characteristics are organized into meaningful groups or patterns of information that alert the nurse to the possibility of an existing patient problem. Usually, the presence of two or three defining characteristics verifies a nursing diagnosis. Occasionally the same descriptors apply to several nursing diagnoses. Pallor, shortness of breath, and expressions of anxiety, for example, are defining characteristics of many nursing diagnoses.

In this text, all NANDA defining characteristics have been included. For some nursing diagnoses, NANDA has further refined the defining characteristics as "major" and "minor." According to NANDA, the major defining characteristics are present 80–100% of the time, while the minor characteristics are present at least 50% of the time (Taxonomy I Revised). As research continues, more major and minor defining characteristics will undoubtedly be identified.

Suggested alternative diagnoses

Suggested alternative diagnoses are other nursing diagnoses that may be considered when identifying the patient's problem. If a review of the definition and defining characteristics indicates that the nursing diagnosis is inaccurate, the nurse may refer to the list of suggested alternative diagnoses for other options. This is particularly helpful for the nurse unfamiliar with the nuances of each nursing diagnosis. Some nursing diagnoses have no suggested alternative diagnoses because of their specificity.

Patient outcomes

Patient outcomes are statements of patient/family behaviors that are measurable, are observable, and denote a desired goal. Patient outcome statements, like all components of the care planning process, are dynamic. Therefore, patient outcomes are frequently changing goals. Some goals are easily achieved and, once accomplished, can be deleted. Others may take longer to achieve and need periodic reevaluation. Measurable patient outcome statements are critical. Without them, the care planning process has no evaluation component.

Not all patient outcomes listed will be appropriate for each patient. The nurse should be realistic when constructing patient outcome statements, because partial behavior change may be the only attainable goal. With shortened length of hospital stay, patient outcomes may be completed after discharge by nurses in the community setting. At time of discharge, the nurse may initiate discussion with the patient to determine patient/family outcomes still requiring completion with referral to appropriate community resources.

Patient outcomes may be selected from this handbook or developed specifically for the patient/family situation. Use as few patient outcomes as are necessary to help the patient achieve his/her goal. Prioritize outcomes with consideration given to length of stay, patient condition, and/or what the patient and family can reasonably accomplish.

Target date

The target date is the estimated date by which the outcome will be accomplished. The date is individualized to the patient, is flexible, and should be reviewed periodically. Target dates are changed as necessary. The target date and its subsequent review help the nurse evaluate the patient's progress toward outcomes.

Documentation interval

The documentation interval designates how often documentation should occur for each outcome. This interval should be determined during initial assessment and may be changed as patient behaviors indicate the completion of a goal (outcome). For example, in the care plan *Fatigue,* the documentation interval for the outcome "Patient demonstrates increasing ability to concentrate," could be specified as "q8 hours." This means that documentation must occur at least every eight hours until the outcome is accomplished.

The evaluation process is incomplete unless a target date and documentation interval accompany each outcome statement. The outcomes, documentation interval, and target date are reviewed for currency and applicability at least daily and are updated as the patient's condition or situation changes.

Nursing interventions

The nursing interventions listed for each care plan include activities performed in the nursing process: assessment diagnosis, planning, interventions, and evaluation. The interventions should be chosen only if they apply to the patient's condition and circumstance. Not every intervention will be appropriate for every patient. For example, it may be necessary to select only a few of the interventions at first and add others later as necessary. The nurse has the option to write interventions that are specific to the patient to ensure an individualized plan of care. In certain instances, "q ___" or "specify plan" is included in the intervention statement as a reminder to individualize the plan. The intervention is not complete without this specificity.

Often, assessment and documentation information is included in an intervention statement. Documentation is essential to quantify nursing actions. This documentation should include the type of nursing intervention, its frequency, and the patient's response. Without this documentation, the patient's progress cannot be evaluated.

Certain interventions require assessment of available laboratory values. Normal ranges for laboratory values vary with the clinical laboratory equipment used in different facilities, and the nurse may need to refer to other resources to evaluate the patient's results.

As the patient's condition changes, interventions may be added, changed, or deleted. Frequent updating of this portion of the care plan is essential.

Clinical Conditions Guide to Nursing Diagnoses

The second part of this handbook is organized to help the nurse select nursing diagnoses when the patient's medical condition is known but the appropriate nursing diagnoses have not yet been established. In this section, medical, surgical, psychiatric, perinatal, and pediatric conditions are listed with suggested nursing diagnoses and their related factors or risk factors. The suggested nursing diagnoses and related factors or risk factors are thought to occur frequently when the particular medical condition is present. When reviewing these lists, the nurse needs to remember that not all of the nursing diagnoses will apply to each patient situation. The nurse should select only those nursing diagnoses that are determined to be applicable from the assessment information collected.

The list of conditions does not include unusual disease conditions, and it may be necessary to refer to a more general title. For example, the patient's medical diagnosis may be scleroderma. Since this condition occurs infrequently, the nurse should look under the general title *Autoimmune Disorders* and review the nursing diagnoses listed there before developing the care plan.

■ How to Create a Nursing Diagnosis Care Plan

The following example shows how to use this book to create a care plan in a specific situation. It illustrates the application of nursing process in the selection of a nursing diagnosis and the subsequent development of a plan of care.

Mrs. B, a seventy-five-year-old female, has been admitted to a surgical unit from the recovery room (postanesthesia recovery) following a hip pinning. Mrs. B's daughter, who is sitting at her mother's bedside, has provided the following history. Mrs. B lives alone in an upstairs apartment, which has been her home for the past twenty-five years. Her husband died ten years ago as a result of Alzheimer's disease. She has many friends and is involved in community affairs at the local senior center where she volunteers her time two days a week for secretarial support. She loves to walk and to ride a bicycle. Her current hospital admission is a result of falling off her bicycle in front of her daughter's house.

Mrs. B's postoperative medical orders include the following:

Foley catheter to gravity drainage

D5 .2% NaCl with KCl 20 mEq to be infused over 8 hours

Advance diet, as tolerated

Vital signs qid

Morphine sulfate 1–2 mg, IV push, q15 minutes until comfortable to a maximum of 10 mg in 1 hour

Morphine sulfate 6–8 mg, IM q3–4 hours, prn pain

Phenergan 25 mg IM q4–6 hours, prn nausea

Monitor intake and output

CBC and electrolytes tomorrow in AM

Overhead trapeze to bed

Turn patient from back to unaffected side q1–2 hours

Pressure-reducing mattress overlay to bed to relieve pressure to bony prominences

Ambulate with assistance in AM and then qid

Turn, cough, and deep breathe at least q2 hours

4:00 PM—The nurse's initial assessment following return from the recovery room indicates that the patient is sleeping comfortably, vital signs are within normal limits, and the operative dressing is dry and intact. Foley catheter is draining clear, amber urine. The IV is infusing at the prescribed rate; skin is warm and dry.

7:00 PM—Mrs. B's daughter has left the bedside to return home.

7:30 PM—The nurse enters Mrs. B's room to check her vital signs and finds Mrs. B attempting to climb out of bed "because I have to go to the bathroom." The nurse reminds Mrs. B that she is in the hospital and has a Foley catheter in place. Mrs. B's responses indicate that she is disoriented to place and time.

The nurse's assessment, of Mrs. B indicates that one possible applicable nursing diagnosis is *Injury: High Risk*. The definition of *Injury: High Risk* is "a state in which the individual is at risk of injury as a result of environmental conditions interacting with the individual's adaptive and defensive resources." The risk factors identified from Mrs. B's assessment data are altered mobility, disorientation, pain medication, and change in environment.

Suggested alternative diagnoses are then considered:

Sensory/Perceptual Alterations

Tissue Perfusion, Altered: Peripheral

Skin Integrity, Impaired: High Risk

After review of the alternatives, the nurse determines that *Injury: High Risk* is the most appropriate nursing diagnosis for Mrs. B.

If the nurse is still unsure which diagnoses are appropriate for Mrs. B, or if the nurse wants to review additional possible nursing diagnoses, the nurse refers to pages 273–274 to look over the *Surgical Conditions* list of possible nursing diagnoses appropriate for *Musculoskeletal Surgery*. The nurse then uses the assessment data to determine which of the nursing diagnoses is appropriate for Mrs. B's care plan.

At this point, the nurse determines the measurable outcomes from the care plan, such as the following:

Patient avoids physical injury.

The outcome is measurable and appropriate for Mrs. B's situation. The documentation interval for the outcome could be q8 hours, and the target date could be 1–2 days after surgery. The target date should be stated as an actual date (e.g., 1/30). The documentation interval and target date should be reviewed at least daily to evaluate appropriateness.

Next, the nurse selects nursing interventions. The following interventions may be selected for Mrs. B's plan of care:

Assess and document patient's motor and/or sensory deficit to determine safety needs of patient. Specify safety needs of patient: ___

Reorient patient to reality and immediate environment when necessary.

Encourage patient to request assistance with activities. Use pressure reduction device, foot cradle, heel and elbow pads to prevent/inhibit skin injury.

All of the aforementioned interventions could be part of Mrs. B's care plan. Once an intervention is no longer applicable, the nurse should delete it from the care plan.

Depending on the assessment data, other nursing diagnoses could apply in this case study. This example demonstrates the process used to develop a care plan using nursing diagnostic statements, patient outcomes, documentation intervals, target dates, and interventions.

■ PLANS OF CARE

Activity Intolerance

Related factors: Anxiety, Arrhythmias, Imbalance between oxygen supply and demand, Acute Pain, Chronic Pain, Weakness/fatigue, Sedentary life-style, Others specific to patient (specify).

Definition: A state in which an individual has insufficient physiologic or psychologic energy to endure or complete required or desired daily activities (NANDA).

■ Defining characteristics

Complaints of fatigue and weakness
Abnormal heart rate or blood pressure in response to activity
Exertional discomfort or dyspnea
EKG changes during activity reflecting arrhythmias or ischemia

■ Suggested alternative diagnoses

Fatigue
Hopelessness
Pain, Chronic

■ Patient outcomes

Patient identifies activities that increase fatigue.
Patient identifies anxiety-producing situations that may contribute to activity intolerance.
Patient participates in required physical activity.
Patient demonstrates ability to intersperse activity with appropriate rest periods.
Patient reports increased comfort while performing activities.
Patient employs safety measures to minimize potential for injury.
Patient verbalizes understanding of need for oxygen, medications, and/or equipment that may increase tolerance for activities.
Patient verbalizes acceptance of limitations in strength and endurance.
Infant demonstrates increasing tolerance for ADLs/activity.
Other outcomes specific to patient (specify).

■ Target date

Specify estimated date of completion.

■ Documentation interval

Specify frequency.

■ Nursing interventions

Assess and document patient's level of tolerance to all activities q ___.

Assess and document presence of increased pulse and respirations, dyspnea, cyanosis, pain, and diaphoresis as indicators of limited tolerance for activity q ___.

Encourage patient to report onset of pain (severity, location, precipitating factors) that may inhibit activity. Document.

Administer pain medications prior to activity.

Encourage patient to request pain medication prior to beginning activity, as necessary.

Encourage patient to report activities that increase fatigue.

Instruct patient/family in ways to identify and decrease anxiety-producing situations.

Instruct patient/family in the use of relaxation techniques (distraction, visualization) during activities.

Instruct patient/family in use of equipment, such as oxygen, during activities.

Plan activities with patient/family that promote independence and minimize fatigue.

    Plan may include:

    Setting small, realistic, attainable goals for patient that increase independence and self-esteem. Specify goals ___.

    Providing rest periods during activities.

    Contracting with patient regarding maintenance of or increase in activity. Contract is ___.

    Providing positive reinforcement for increased activity.

    Assisting with activity, as needed. Specify assistance needed.

    Providing safe environment by removing obstacles from ambulation area.

    Keeping frequently used objects within easy reach of patient.

    Including family in assisting patient with activities, as appropriate (specify).

Plan care for the infant/child to minimize the oxygen needs of the body:

    Provide adequate rest.

    Anticipate needs for food, water, comfort, and holding and stimulation, which will prevent unnecessary crying.

    Minimize anxiety and stress.

    Monitor activity level and exercise tolerance.

    Prevent hyperthermia and hypothermia.

    Avoid environments low in oxygen concentration, e.g., high altitudes, unpressurized airplanes.

    Prevent infection.

Other interventions specific to patient (specify).

Activity Intolerance: High Risk

Risk factors: History of previous intolerance, Deconditioned status, Presence of circulatory/respiratory problems, Inexperience with the activity, Others specific to patient (specify).

Definition: State in which an individual is at risk of experiencing insufficient physiologic or psychologic energy to endure or complete required or desired daily activities (NANDA).

■ Suggested alternative diagnoses

Disuse Syndrome: High risk

■ Patient outcomes

Patient identifies risk factors that interfere with completing daily activities.
Patient describes plan for adapting to obstacles that inhibit activity.
Patient completes desired/required daily activities.
Patient uses safety measures to minimize potential for injury during activity.
Other outcomes specific to patient (specify).

■ Target date	■ Documentation interval
Specify estimated date of completion.	Specify frequency.

■ Nursing interventions

Explore with patient the specific consequences of inactivity.
Continually assess patient for development of actual intolerance to activity.
Identify the obstacles to activity.
Develop a realistic plan for adapting to patient's limitations.
Enlist family in efforts to support and encourage the patient's completion of activities.
Other interventions specific to patient (specify).

Adjustment, Impaired

Related factors: Assault to self-esteem, Impaired cognition, Inadequate support systems, Incomplete grieving, Necessity for major life-style/behavior changes secondary to ___, Pattern of dependence, Sensory overload, Altered locus of control, Others specific to patient (specify).

Definition: The state in which an individual is unable to modify his/her life-style/behavior in a manner consistent with a change in health status (NANDA).

■ **Defining characteristics**

Major	*Minor*
Verbalizes nonacceptance of health status change	Lack of movement toward independence
Inability to problem solve or set goals	Extended period of shock, disbelief, or anger regarding health status change
	Lack of future-oriented thinking

■ **Suggested alternative diagnoses**

Coping, Ineffective Individual
Grieving, Dysfunctional
Health Maintenance, Altered
Hopelessness
Noncompliance (specify)
Powerlessness
Self-esteem, Low: Chronic
Therapeutic Regimen Management, Ineffective Individual

■ **Patient outcomes**

Patient acknowledges importance of life-style/behavior changes.
Patient verbalizes feelings about required life-style/behavior changes.
Patient identifies obstacles that hinder life-style/behavior changes.
Patient identifies personal strengths that will promote life-style/behavior changes.
Patient acknowledges value of independent behaviors.
Patient follows agreed-upon plan.
Patient demonstrates decreased anxiety and fear in independent activities.
Other outcomes specific to patient (specify).

■ **Target date**	■ **Documentation interval**
Specify estimated date of completion.	Specify frequency.

■ **Nursing interventions**

Assess extent of patient's inability to solve problems and/or set goals.

Provide a nonjudgmental environment in which patient/family can share concerns/anxieties/fears.

Include patient/family in a multidisciplinary conference to establish a plan of care. Plan may include:

Assisting patient/family in reviewing necessary life-style/behavior changes and selecting one as an initial goal.

Assisting patient to identify personal strengths that will help patient to achieve goals.

Assisting patient to identify obstacles that hinder life-style/behavior changes.

Setting realistic goals/limits. Prioritize goals/limits, and establish target dates.

Providing continuity of patient care throughout patient assignment and use of care plan.

Encourage and support patient's demonstration of desirable behavior changes.

Encourage patient to meet/discuss with patients in similar situations to learn new ways to cope and to decrease isolation and fear.

Refer patient to community agencies and/or support groups.

Other interventions specific to patient (specify).

Airway Clearance, Ineffective

Related factors: Decreased energy/fatigue, Trauma, Tracheobronchial infection, Tracheobronchial obstruction, Tracheobronchial secretions, Perceptive/cognitive impairment, Others specific to patient (specify).

Definition: A state in which an individual is unable to clear secretions or obstructions from the respiratory tract to maintain airway patency (NANDA).

■ Defining characteristics

Abnormal breath sounds, such as rales, rhonchi
Changes in rate or depth of respiration
Tachypnea
Cough: effective or ineffective, with or without sputum
Cyanosis
Dyspnea

■ Suggested alternative diagnosis

Aspiration: High Risk

■ Patient outcomes

Patient is able to expectorate secretions effectively.
Patient has patent airway.
Pulmonary function is within normal limits for patient.
Patient is able to describe plan for care at home.
Other outcomes specific to patient (specify).

■ Target date   ■ Documentation interval

Specify estimated date of completion.   Specify frequency.

■ Nursing interventions

Auscultate anterior and posterior chest q ___ to evaluate airway clearance.

Assess and document effectiveness of prescribed medications q ___.

Assess and document effectiveness of oxygen administration q ___.

Observe and document color, consistency, and amount of sputum.

Assess and document trends in arterial blood gases, and notify physician of abnormalities.

Correlate all assessment data (patient sensorium, breath sounds, respiratory pattern, ABGs, sputum production), document, and report any changes.

Consult with physician concerning need for percussion and/or supportive equipment.

Explain proper use of supportive equipment (oxygen, suction, spirometer, IPPB).

Confer with respiratory therapist as needed.

Suction the nasopharynx/oropharynx to remove secretions q ___.

Suction q ___. (Be sure to hyperoxygenate with ambu bag before and after suctioning ET tube or trach.)

Maintain adequate hydration to decrease viscosity of secretions.

Encourage physical activity to promote movement of secretions.

Inform patient before initiating procedures to lower anxiety and increase sense of control.

Inform patient and family that smoking is prohibited in room.

Instruct patient in coughing and deep-breathing techniques, which facilitate removal of secretions.

Instruct patient and family in plan for care at home (medications, hydration, nebulization, equipment, postural drainage, signs and symptoms of complications, community resources).

Other interventions specific to patient (specify).

Anxiety

Related factors: Unconscious conflict about essential values/goals of life, Threat to self-concept, Threat of death, Threat to or change in health status, Threat to or change in role functioning, Threat to or change in environment, Threat to or change in interaction patterns, Situational/maturational crises, Interpersonal transmission/contagion, Unmet needs, Others specific to patient (specify).

Definition: A vague, uneasy feeling whose source is often nonspecific or unknown to the individual (NANDA).

■ Defining characteristics

Increased tension	Anxiousness
Apprehension	Sympathetic stimulation
Painful and persistent increased helplessness	Cardiovascular excitation
	Superficial vasoconstriction
Uncertainty	Pupil dilation
Fearfulness	Restlessness
Regret	Insomnia
Overexcitement	Glancing about
Becoming rattled	Poor eye contact
Distress	Trembling/hand tremors
Becoming jittery	Extraneous movement (foot shuffling,
Feelings of inadequacy	hand/arm movements)
Shakiness	Facial tension
Fear of unspecific consequences	Voice quivering
Expressed concerns about change in life events	Focus on self
	Increased wariness
Worry	Increased perspiration

■ Suggested alternative diagnoses

Coping, Ineffective Individual
Fear
Post-Trauma Response
Rape-Trauma Syndrome: Silent Reaction

■ Patient outcomes

Patient identifies those symptoms that are indicators of own anxiety.
Patient uses anxiety-reducing techniques.
Patient demonstrates ability to continue necessary activities even though anxiety persists.
Patient reports reduction in anxiety.
Patient reports a decrease in somatic complaints.
Patient demonstrates ability to focus on new knowledge and skills.
Other outcomes specific to patient (specify).

■ **Target date**   ■ **Documentation interval**

Specify estimated date of completion.   Specify frequency.

■ **Nursing interventions**

Assess and document patient's level of anxiety q ___.

Encourage patient to verbalize thoughts and feelings to externalize anxiety.

Help patient identify events that have precipitated anxiety in the past.

Explore with patient techniques that have, and have not, reduced anxiety in the past. Specify ___.

Help patient to focus on the present situation as a means of identifying coping mechanisms needed to reduce anxiety.

Reassure patient during interactions by touch and empathetic verbal and nonverbal exchanges, encourage patient to express anger and irritation, and allow patient to cry.

Reduce excessive stimulation by providing a quiet environment, limited contact with others if necessary, and limited use of caffeine and other stimulants.

Suggest alternative methods of reducing anxiety that are acceptable to patient. Specify ___.

Provide diversion through television, radio, games, and occupational therapies to reduce anxiety and expand focus.

Provide positive reinforcement when patient is able to continue ADLs and other activities necessary to progress to optimal wellness.

Develop teaching plan with realistic goals, including need for repetition, encouragement, and praise of the tasks learned. Specify plan ___.

Other interventions specific to patient (specify).

Aspiration: High Risk

Risk factors: Reduced level of consciousness, Depressed cough and gag reflexes, Presence of tracheostomy or endotracheal tube, Incomplete lower esophageal sphincter, Gastrointestinal tubes, Tube feedings, Medication administration, Increased intragastric pressure, Increased gastric residual, Decreased gastrointestinal motility, Impaired swallowing, Delayed gastric emptying, Facial/oral/neck surgery or trauma, Wired jaws, Hindered elevation of upper body, Others specific to patient (specify).

Definition: The state in which an individual is at risk for entry of gastrointestinal secretions, oropharyngeal secretions, or solids or fluids into tracheobronchial passages (NANDA).

■ Suggested alternative diagnoses

Airway Clearance, Ineffective
Self-Care Deficit: Feeding
Swallowing, Impaired

■ Patient outcomes

Patient demonstrates increased improvement in swallowing.
Patient swallows independently without choking.
Patient tolerates oral intake and secretions without aspiration.
Patient tolerates enteral feedings without aspiration.
Other outcomes specific to patient (specify).

■ Target date   ■ Documentation interval

Specify estimated date of completion.   Specify frequency.

■ Nursing interventions

Evaluate patient for potential aspiration, including LOC, tube placement, handling of secretions.

Monitor tube feeding residual q ___.

Have suction catheter available at bedside, and suction during meals as needed.

Place patient in semi- or high-Fowler's position when eating whenever possible.

Crush medications to facilitate swallowing.

Provide positive reinforcement for attempts to swallow independently.

Use syringe, if necessary, when feeding patient to facilitate swallowing.

Request occupational therapy consultation.

Involve family during patient's ingestion of food and meals:
> Review signs and symptoms of aspiration and preventive measures.
> Instruct family in feeding/swallowing techniques.
> Evaluate family's comfort level.
> Provide support and reassurance.

For patients unable to sit upright, place on side, and elevate head of bed as much as possible during and after feeding.

Verify placement of enteral tube prior to feeding and giving medications.

Check gastric residual prior to feeding and giving medications.

Instruct patient in use of Yankauer suction for removal of secretions.

Vary consistency of foods to identify those foods more easily tolerated.

Allow patient time to swallow.

Assess patient's lung sounds q___ before and after feeding, before and after giving medication; document any adventitious sounds.

Report any change in color of lung secretions that resembles food or feeding intake.

Other interventions specific to patient (specify).

Body Image Disturbance

Related factors: Cultural or spiritual beliefs, Eating disorders (specify), Surgery, Pregnancy, Situational crisis (specify), Psychologic impairment (specify), Chronic illness, Chronic pain, Treatment side-effects, Congenital defects, Others specific to patient (specify).

Definition: Viewing oneself differently as a result of actual or perceived changes in body structure or function.

■ Defining characteristics

Verbal response to actual or perceived change in structure or function[1]

Expressing negative feelings about body
Expressing feelings of helplessness, hopelessness, or powerlessness
Reporting changes in life-style
Refusal to accept change
Preoccupation with change or loss
Verbalizing fear of rejection by or reaction of others
Focusing on past strengths, function, or appearance
Extension of body boundary to incorporate environmental objects
Personalization of body part or loss by name
Emphasis on remaining strengths and heightened achievement
Depersonalization of part or loss by impersonal pronouns

Nonverbal response to actual or perceived change in structure or function[1]

Not touching body part
Showing reluctance to touch or look at affected body part
Actual change in structure or function
Missing body part
Hiding or overexposing body part (intentional or unintentional)
Change in ability to estimate spatial relationship of body to environment
Trauma to nonfunctioning part
Change in social involvement
Not looking at body part

■ Suggested alternative diagnoses

Growth and Development, Altered
Nutrition, Altered: More Than Body Requirements
Rape-Trauma Syndrome
Self-Esteem Disturbance

■ **Patient outcomes**

Patient identifies personal strengths.
Patient acknowledges the actual change in body appearance.
Patient acknowledges impact of situation on existing personal relationships and life-style.
Patient maintains close personal relationships.
Patient expresses willingness to consider life-style change.
Patient expresses willingness to use suggested resources on discharge.
Patient describes actual change in function.
Other outcomes specific to patient (specify).

■ **Target date**	■ **Documentation interval**
Specify estimated date of completion.	Specify frequency.

■ **Nursing interventions**

Encourage patient to verbalize consequences of physical and emotional changes that have influenced self-concept.
Encourage patient to maintain usual daily grooming routine.
Encourage patient to wear clothing to enhance physical and emotional self-esteem.
Encourage patient to verbalize concerns about close personal relationships.
Actively listen to patient/family, and acknowledge reality of concerns about treatments, progress, and prognosis.
Encourage patient/family to air feelings and to grieve.
Provide care in a nonjudgmental manner, maintaining the patient's privacy and dignity.
Assist patient in identifying personal strengths.
Help patient identify alternative behaviors that are congruent with a change in personal relationships, life-style, and/or role performance.
Develop a plan of care with patient/family that identifies coping mechanisms and personal strengths and acknowledges limitations. Specify plan.
Assess need for assistance from social services department for planning care with patient/family.
Offer to make initial phone call to appropriate community resources for patient/family.
Other interventions specific to patient (specify).

---

[1]Must be present to justify diagnosis.

Body Temperature, Altered: High Risk

Risk factors: Altered metabolic rate, Dehydration, Exposure to extremes in environmental temperatures, Extremes of age, Extremes of weight, Inability to perspire, Inappropriate clothing, Medications (specify), Low birth weight, Immaturity of newborn's temperature-regulating system, Inactivity, Vigorous activity, Sedation, Illness or trauma affecting temperature regulation, Others specific to patient (specify).

Definition: The state in which the individual is at risk for failure to maintain body temperature within normal range (NANDA).

■ **Suggested alternative diagnoses**

Home Maintenance Management, Impaired
Hyperthermia
Hypothermia

■ **Patient outcomes**

Temperature remains within normal limits for patient.
Patient/family describes adaptive measures to minimize fluctuations in body temperature.
Patient/family reports early signs/symptoms of hypothermia/hyperthermia.
Other outcomes specific to patient (specify).

■ Target date	■ Documentation interval
Specify estimated date of completion.	Specify frequency.

■ **Nursing interventions**

Monitor temperature q ___.
Maintain stable environmental temperature.
Assess patient for early signs and symptoms of hypothermia/hyperthermia.
Instruct patient/family in measures to minimize temperature fluctuations.

Hypothermia	*Hyperthermia*
Wear adequate clothing.	Remove excess clothing.
Maintain adequate nourishment.	Lose weight, if obese.
Maintain stable environmental temperature.	Maintain stable environmental temperature.
Increase activity.	Limit activity on hot days.
Limit alcohol intake.	Drink adequate fluids.
Bathe in warm room, away from drafts.	

Instruct patient/family to recognize and report early signs and symptoms of hypothermia/hyperthermia:

Hypothermia	*Hyperthermia*
Temperature of less than 95° F	Weakness
Impaired ability to think	Headache
Reduced pulse and respiration	Increased pulse
Hypertension	Dry skin
Disorientation/confusion	Irritability
Drowsiness	Increased temperature
Apathy	Temperature above ___
Skin hard and cold to touch	
Cold, hard abdomen that feels like marble	
Hypoglycemia	

Evaluate home environment for factors that may alter body temperature.
Have social services meet with patient/family prior to discharge.
Other interventions specific to patient (specify).

Bowel Incontinence

Related factors: Decreased awareness of need to defecate, Loss of sphincter control, Others specific to patient (specify).

Definition: A state in which an individual experiences a change in normal bowel habits characterized by involuntary passage of stool (NANDA).

■ Defining characteristics

Involuntary passage of stool

■ Suggested alternative diagnoses

Diarrhea

■ Patient outcomes

Patient is free of skin irritation to perianal area.
Patient has fewer incontinent episodes.
Patient regains voluntary control of defecation.
Other outcomes specific to patient (specify).

■ Target date	■ Documentation interval
Specify estimated date of completion.	Specify frequency.

■ Nursing interventions

Document frequency of incontinent episodes.
Assess condition of perianal skin after each episode of incontinence. Document q ___.
Protect patient's skin from involuntary stool (for example, use protective pad and ointments, frequently change bed linen).
Provide bedpan or assist to commode q ___.
Obtain order from physician to institute bowel-training program. (Program may include bulk-forming laxative; rectal suppository q day; digital stimulation; scheduled use of bedpan, commode, or bathroom.)
Provide care in an accepting, nonjudgmental manner.
Provide privacy for patient.
Other interventions specific to patient (specify).

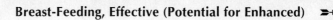

Breast-Feeding, Effective *(Potential for Enhanced)*

Related factors: Basic breast-feeding knowledge, Normal breast structure, Normal infant oral structure, Infant gestational age of more than 34 weeks, Supportive resources, Maternal confidence, Others specific to patient (specify).

Definition: The state in which a mother-infant dyad/family exhibits adequate proficiency and satisfaction with breast-feeding process (NANDA).

■ **Defining characteristics**

Major	*Minor*
Ability of mother to position infant at breast to promote a successful latch-on response	Signs and/or symptoms of oxytocin release (letdown or milk-ejection reflex)
Contentment of infant after feeding	Adequate infant elimination patterns for age
Regular and sustained suckling/ swallowing at breast	Eagerness of infant to nurse
Appropriate infant weight patterns for age	Maternal verbalization of satisfaction with the breast-feeding process
Effective mother-infant communication patterns (infant cues, maternal interpretation or response)	

■ **Suggested alternative diagnoses**

None

■ **Patient outcomes**

Mother and infant maintain effective breast-feeding for as long as planned.
Other outcomes specific to patient (specify).

■ **Target date**	■ **Documentation interval**
Specify estimated date of completion.	Specify frequency.

■ **Nursing interventions**

Early postpartum

Establish correct breast-feeding technique.

Promote maternal confidence by providing positive feedback.

Instruct mother in usual breast-feeding norms, e.g., increased frequency of nursing in first weeks of life, baby's elimination patterns, uterine contractions during nursing.

Discuss breast-feeding schedule, usually a "demand" time every 1 1/2 to 3 hours. Instruct mother to rest during/between feedings.

Provide anticipatory guidance for potential problems such as maternal fatigue; breast engorgement; sore, cracked nipples; inadequate milk supply; multiple births.

Discuss ways to enhance milk supply:

    Drinking plenty of fluids.

    Getting enough rest.

    Nursing frequently.

    Using alternate breast at start of each feeding.

Provide written materials for continued self-care at home.

Make referrals to appropriate community resources, such as Nursing Mothers' Council, La Leche League, other nursing mothers.

Confirm that infant has follow-up appointment with pediatrician.

Home care

Assess breast-feeding technique within first 5–7 days after birth.

Promote maternal confidence by providing encouragement, praise, and reassurance.

Discuss setting priorities that:

    Increase mother's rest.

    Minimize care of house.

    Delegate meal preparation.

Encourage mother to enlist/request available resources for assistance, e.g., family, public health nurse, pediatrician, La Leche League, Nursing Mothers' Council.

Explore mother's breast-feeding plans, e.g., duration, return to work, introduction of solid foods, weaning; provide anticipatory guidance.

Discuss impact of breast-feeding on family dynamics.

Provide instruction regarding breast engorgement, cracked and sore nipples, manual expression, infant appetite spurts, supplemental feedings.

Confirm infant's elimination pattern.

Discuss mother's need to check with physician prior to taking any medication while breast-feeding.

Other interventions specific to patient (specify).

Breast-Feeding, Ineffective

Related factors: Inadequate sucking reflex in infant; Maternal anxiety or ambivalence, Interruption in breast-feeding, Nonsupportive partner/family, Prematurity, Infant anomaly, Maternal breast anomaly, Previous breast surgery, Previous history of breast-feeding failure, Infant receiving supplemental feedings with artificial nipple, Knowledge deficit, Others specific to patients (specify).

Definition: The state in which mother, infant, or child experiences dissatisfaction or difficulty with the breast-feeding process (NANDA).

■ **Defining characteristics**

Major	*Minor*
Unsatisfactory breast-feeding process	Actual or perceived inadequate milk supply
	Inability of infant to latch onto maternal breast correctly
	No observable signs of oxytocin release
	Observable signs of inadequate infant intake
	Nonsustained suckling at the breast
	Insufficient emptying of each breast per feeding
	Persistence of sore nipples beyond the first week of breast-feeding
	Insufficient opportunity for suckling at the breast
	Fussiness and crying within the first hour after breast-feeding
	Unresponsiveness to other comfort measures
	Arching and crying at the breast
	Resistance to latching on

■ **Suggested alternative diagnoses**

Infant Feeding Pattern, Ineffective

■ **Patient outcomes**

Baby gains ___ grams/day or ___ grams/week.
Mother states satisfaction with breast-feeding.
Mother describes increasing confidence with breast-feeding.

■ **Target date**   ■ **Documentation interval**

Specify estimated date of completion.   Specify frequency.

■ **Nursing interventions**

Assess mother's breast-feeding techniques and infant's ability to latch on and suck effectively.

Instruct mother in breast-feeding techniques that increase her skill in feeding infant. Consider relaxation techniques, comfortable positioning, stimulating root reflex, stimulating infant to continue to feed, alternating breasts, and gradual increase of time on breast.

Reinforce successful behaviors.

Instruct mother in need for adequate rest and intake of fluids.

Schedule rest periods as needed.

Offer food and fluids to mother during day and evening prior to breast-feeding times.

Instruct mother in breast-pumping techniques to maintain milk supply during interruptions or delays in infant suckling reflex.

Schedule infant activities to conserve energy prior to breast-feeding.

Use ___ nipples.

Recognize "time-out" behaviors in premature infant.

Have mother express enough milk to relieve engorgement, allowing nipples to evert.

Increase number of nursings on demand for a crying, wakeful infant. Increase number of scheduled nursings for the sleepy infant of low birth weight.

Provide privacy for mother and infant.

Make referrals to appropriate community resources, such as Nursing Mothers' Council, La Leche League, Public Health Department.

Other interventions specific to patient (specify).

Breast-Feeding, Interrupted

Related factors: Maternal or infant illness, Prematurity, Maternal obligations outside the home, Engorgement, Sore/cracked nipples, Maternal medications that are contraindicated for the infant, Abrupt weaning of infant.

Definition: A break in the continuity of the breast-feeding process as a result of inability or inadvisability to put baby to breast for feeding (NANDA).

■ **Defining characteristics**

Major	*Minor*
Infant does not receive nourishment at the breast for some or all of feedings	Maternal desire to maintain lactation and provide (or eventually provide) breast milk for her infant's nutritional needs
	Separation of mother and infant
	Lack of knowledge regarding expression and storage of breast milk

■ **Suggested alternative diagnoses**

Breast-feeding, Ineffective

■ **Patient outcomes**

Mother chooses and demonstrates preferred technique for expression of milk.
Mother describes safe storage techniques for expressed milk.
Baby receives mother's milk.
Maternal lactation is maintained for as long as desired.
Baby latches on and sucks effectively at the breast.
Mother and baby maintain effective breast-feeding for as long as planned.
Other outcomes specific to patient (specify).

■ **Target date**

Specify estimated date of completion.

■ **Documentation interval**

Specify frequency.

■ **Nursing interventions**

Provide information about lactation, breast milk expression (manual and electric pump), collection, and storage.

Display/demonstrate variety of breast pumps, providing information about costs, effectiveness, and availability of each.

Instruct mother in chosen breast-pumping method.

Provide anticipatory guidance for potential problems (e.g., engorgement, pain, leaking, diminished milk production, feelings of disappointment/anger, depression, guilt, inadequacy).

Establish support network to ensure that mother has help with day-to-day lactation/breast-feeding problems as they occur.

Assist mother in setting realistic goals for herself.

Assess family's ability to support lactation/breast-feeding plan and cope with life-style changes.

Assist mother and premature infant with transition to breast:

  Confirm readiness for transition to breast (infant's stability when outside the isolette, infant's coordination of sucking/swallowing/breathing, mother's willingness to try).

  Provide privacy.

  Encourage skin-to-skin contact for mother and infant, using cover blanket over infant to maintain body temperature.

  Position baby with one hand supporting head and other free to manipulate breast; ear, shoulder, and hips of infant should be aligned so that mother's nipples do not become sore.

  Provide mother with written/pictorial references.

  Time at breast will be longer than at bottle, but not to point of infant's exhaustion; once latched on, allow infant to nurse until baby stops sucking and swallowing. Switch baby to other breast and repeat until suck/swallow stops, then switch back.

  Help infant open mouth wider.

  Consider a feeding flow sheet to facilitate assessment: document infant's state, oxygen needs, positioning, time at breast, total nursing time, daily weight, stool pattern.

Assist working mother to maintain lactation and effective breast-feeding:

  A few days before mother's return to work, introduce baby to bottle (someone other than mother, when mother is not present, when baby is hungry, in a different place than usual place for breast-feeding).

  Develop schedule for expression and storage of milk at work.

  Provide information to enhance milk volume (adequate rest, regular expression of milk, increase mother's intake of fluid, especially toward the end of the work week).

  Educate infant caretaker (storage and thawing of milk, no bottle feedings in the 2 hours prior to mother's return home).

If abrupt weaning is necessary, assist mother to:
  Manage breast discomfort.
  Introduce bottle feeding.
  Verbalize feelings about sudden change in plans.
Other interventions specific to patient (specify).

Breathing Pattern, Ineffective

Related factors: Anxiety, Decreased energy/fatigue, Perception/cognitive impairment, Musculoskeletal impairment, Chronic or acute pain, Neuromuscular paralysis/weakness, Others specific to patient (specify).

Definition: The state in which an individual's inhalation and/or exhalation pattern does not enable adequate pulmonary inflation or emptying (NANDA).

■ Defining characteristics

Pursed lip breathing/prolonged expiratory phase
Dyspnea
Tachypnea
Cyanosis
Fremitus
Cough
Assumption of 3-point position

Shortness of breath
Change in depth of respirations
Abnormal blood gases
Increased anterior-posterior diameter
Use of accessory muscles
Altered chest excursion
Premature infant
Nasal flaring

■ Suggested alternative diagnoses

None

■ Patient outcomes

Patient requests breathing assistance when needed.
Patient demonstrates effective breathing pattern.
Patient demonstrates optimal breathing while on mechanical ventilator.
Pulmonary function is within normal limits for patient.
Patient/family is able to describe plan for care at home.
Other outcomes specific to patient (specify).

■ Target date

Specify estimated date of completion.

■ Documentation interval

Specify frequency.

■ Nursing interventions

Assess and document presence or absence of breath sounds (anterior and posterior), noting rales, rhonchi, and diminished breath sounds q ___.

Assess and document respiratory pattern, including rate, depth, and rhythm q ___.

Assess and document cyanosis q ___.

Position for optimal breathing (specify).

Maintain low-flow oxygen by nasal cannula, mask, hood, or tent. Specify flow rate: ___.

Assess and document effect of medication on respiratory status.

Assess and document location and extent of crepitus over rib cage.

Correlate all assessment data (patient sensorium, breath sounds, respiratory pattern, ABGs, sputum, effect of medications), document, and report any changes.

Instruct patient to notify nurse at onset of ineffective breathing pattern.

Reassure patient during periods of respiratory distress.

Encourage slow abdominal breathing during periods of respiratory distress.

Have patient turn, cough, and deep breathe q ___.

Give pain medications to allow optimal respiratory pattern according to the following schedule (specify schedule): ___.

Inform patient and family that smoking is prohibited in room.

Inform patient before beginning intended procedures to lower anxiety and increase sense of control.

Instruct patient in relaxation techniques to improve breathing pattern. Specify.

Synchronize patient's breathing pattern with ventilator rate.

Observe and document bilateral chest expansion of patient on ventilator.

Confer with respiratory therapist to ensure adequate functioning of mechanical ventilator.

Instruct patient and family in plan for care at home (medications, supportive equipment, signs and symptoms of reportable complications, community resources).

Other interventions specific to patient (specify).

Cardiac Output, Decreased

Related factors: Cardiac anomaly (specify), Drug toxicity, Dysfunctional electrical conduction, Hypovolemia, Increased ventricular workload, Ventricular ischemia, Ventricular damage, Ventricular restriction, Others specific to patient (specify).

Definition: A state in which the blood pumped by an individual's heart is sufficiently reduced that it is inadequate to meet the needs of the body's tissues (NANDA).

■ **Defining characteristics**

Major	*Minor*
Color changes in skin and mucous membranes	Change in mental status
	Shortness of breath
Restlessness	Syncope
Dyspnea	Vertigo
Decreased peripheral pulses	Edema
Cold, clammy skin	Cough
Jugular vein distention	Frothy sputum
Rales	Gallop rhythm
Oliguria	Weakness
Orthopnea	
Variations in blood pressure readings	
Arrhythmias	
Fatigue	

■ **Suggested alternative diagnoses**

None

■ **Patient outcomes**

Patient maintains hemodynamic stability. Specify normal limits for blood pressure, pulse, pulse pressure, respirations, and hemodynamic parameters.
Patient reports a decrease in severity and frequency of pain.
Patient demonstrates increasing tolerance for physical activity.
Patient describes the required diet, medications, activity, and limitations.
Patient identifies reportable signs and symptoms of worsening condition.
Other outcomes specific to patient (specify).

■ **Target date**	■ **Documentation interval**
Specify estimated date of completion.	Specify frequency.

■ **Nursing interventions**

Correlate baseline vital signs with current vital signs, and assess for changes in blood pressure, pulse (rate, rhythm, quality), and respirations and hemodynamic parameters.

Assess and document dysrhythmias q ___. Correlate effects of laboratory values, oxygen, medications, activity, anxiety, and/or pain on the dysrhythmia.

Assess and document patient's tolerance to activity by noting onset of shortness of breath, pain, palpitations, or dizziness.

Correlate patient's blood pressure with blood pressure medications administered. Withhold blood pressure medications when there is a drop in blood pressure, and notify physician.

Confer with physician regarding parameters for administering/withholding blood pressure medications.

Evaluate blood pressure, presence of cyanosis, respiratory status, peripheral perfusion, mental status, and urine output. Document findings.

Maintain patient's appropriate/required activity level. Specify.

Change patient's position to flat/Trendelenberg when blood pressure is in a range lower than normal for patient. Document patient's response to position change.

Evaluate patient for fluid overload by assessing presence of dependent edema, weight gain, and decreased urine output. Auscultate lungs for adventitious sounds. Document.

Instruct patient in maintenance of accurate intake and output.

For sudden, severe, or prolonged hypotension, establish intravenous access for administration of intravenous fluids and/or medications to raise blood pressure.

Instruct patient to report and describe palpitations and pain onset, duration, precipitating factors, site, quality, and intensity.

Explain purpose of administering oxygen per nasal cannula or mask.

Instruct patient on use, dose, frequency, and side-effects of medications. Document instruction in nurse's notes.

Instruct patient/family in plan for care at home, including activity limitations, diet restrictions, use of therapeutic equipment, and reportable signs and symptoms.

Provide information on stress-reduction techniques such as biofeedback, progressive muscle relaxation, meditation, exercise.

Other interventions specific to patient (specify).

Caregiver Role Strain (Actual/High Risk)

Related factors/risk factors: *Pathophysiological:* Illness severity of the care receiver, Addiction or codependency, Premature birth/congenital defect, Discharge of family member with significant home care needs, Caregiver health impairment, Unpredictable illness course or instability in the care receiver's health; *Developmental:* Caregiver not developmentally ready for caregiver role, e.g., young adult needing to provide care for a middle-aged parent, Developmental delay or retardation of the care receiver or caregiver; *Psychosocial:* Caregiver is female, Caregiver is spouse, Caregiver's marginal coping patterns, Past history of poor relationship between caregiver and care receiver, Marginal family adaptation or dysfunction prior to the caregiving situation, Psychological or cognitive problems in care receiver, Care receiver exhibits deviant, bizarre behavior; *Situational:* Presence of abuse or violence, Presence of situational stressors that normally affect families, such as significant loss, disaster or crisis, poverty or economic vulnerability, major life events, e.g., birth, hospitalization, leaving home, returning home, marriage, divorce, employment, retirement, death, Duration of required caregiving, Inadequate physical environment for providing care, e.g., housing, transportation, community services, equipment, Family/caregiver isolation, Lack of respite and recreation for caregiver, Inexperience with/lack of knowledge of caregiving skills, Caregiver's competing role commitments, Complexity/amount of caregiving tasks.

Definition (Actual): A caregiver's felt difficulty in performing the family caregiver role (NANDA).

Definition (High risk): A caregiver is vulnerable for felt difficulty in performing the family caregiver role (NANDA).

■ Defining characteristics

80% of caregivers report one or more of the following defining characteristics:
   Do not have sufficient resources to provide the care needed
   Find it hard to perform specific caregiving activities
   Worry about the care receiver's health and emotional state, having to put the
      care receiver in an institution, and who will care for the care receiver if
      something should happen to the caregiver
   Feel that caregiving interferes with other important roles in their lives
   Feel loss because the care receiver is a different person than before caregiving
      began or, in the case of a child, that the care receiver was never the child the
      caregiver expected
   Feel family conflict around issues of providing care
   Feel stress or nervousness in their relationship with the care receiver
   Feel depressed

■ **Suggested alternative diagnoses**

Coping, Ineffective Family: Compromised
Coping, Ineffective Family: Disabling
Family Processes, Altered
Parental Role Conflict
Role Performance, Altered

■ **Patient outcomes**

Caregiver acknowledges impact of situation on existing life-style/role performance.
Caregiver identifies personal strengths, social supports, and community resources.
Caregiver expresses willingness to identify and use available resources and social
    supports.
Caregiver expresses increased ability to cope with changes in family structure and
    dynamics.
Caregiver balances competing family and personal needs.
Caregiver ensures provision of appropriate level of care.
Care receiver obtains appropriate assistance/care through caregiver's efforts.
Other outcomes specific to caregiver (specify).

■ **Target date**   ■ **Documentation interval**

Specify estimated date of completion.   Specify frequency.

■ **Nursing interventions**

Acknowledge that the work of the caregiver is both physical and mental and includes (Bowers, 1987):

Anticipatory caregiving (making decisions based on possible future needs of care receiver, e.g., place of residence).

Preventive caregiving (taking action to prevent illness, injury, or complications, e.g., altering the physical environment, preparing meals).

Supervisory caregiving (arranging for and monitoring care, e.g., making appointments, arranging transportation, communicating with health professionals).

Instrumental caregiving (direct, hands-on care).

Protective caregiving (protecting care receiver from threats to self-image, identity, and change in relationship with caregiver).

Arrange for parent(s) of chronically ill child to receive training in areas of child development and education, and compliance-related behavior problems.

Facilitate coping and adjustment by teaching caregiver and care receiver how to (Chilman, 1988):

Deal with pain, incapacitation, and illness-related symptoms.

Deal with hospital environment and disease-related treatments/procedures.

Establish and maintain workable relationships with the health care team.

Assess family's adjustment and coping; make referrals as needed for counseling and support during times of stress or crisis.

Facilitate family's adjustment to illness of family member by assisting them to (Chilman, 1988):

Maintain a sense of mastery over their lives.

Grieve for the loss of pre-illness family identity.

Move toward acceptance of changes.

Pull together during short-term crisis.

Develop a flexibility regarding future goals.

Assist caregiver to identify problems or concerns with caregiving (e.g., lack of knowledge/skill/emotional readiness for caregiving, lack of social support, financial burden, caregiver response to care receiver's mental deterioration, disruptive behavior, impaired social functioning, increasing need for physical care).

Explore with caregiver/care receiver past and current closeness, shared activities, and confiding in one another as indications of emotional investment and commitment to the role.

Promote self-care by care receiver, as appropriate, to encourage relief for caregiver (Schainen, 1991).

Assess caregiver for signs of increasing role strain (e.g., depression, anxiety, increased use/abuse of alcohol/drugs, frustration, helplessness, sleeplessness, lowered morale, physical and/or emotional exhaustion, and personal health problems).

Assess care receiver for signs of emotional and/or physical neglect or abuse, and if present, report to appropriate authorities.

Explore with caregiver the possibility of institutional care (now or in the future) and feelings associated with institutionalization.

Develop a plan of care with caregiver that identifies coping mechanisms, personal strengths, social supports, and acknowledged limitations. Consider including the following:

Caregiver education and training groups.

Self-help and mutual support groups for information, advocacy, and emotional support.

Referrals for assistance with preventive, supervisory, and instrumental caregiving (e.g., VNA, respite care, hospice care, day treatment, secondary caregivers).

Assistance with household tasks.

Family therapy.

Other interventions specific to caregiver (specify).

Communication, Impaired: Verbal

Related factors: Acute confusion, Aphasia, Developmental disability, Psychologic impairment (specify), Inability to speak or speak clearly, Intubation, Primary language other than English, Tracheostomy, Others specific to patient (specify).

Definition: The state in which an individual experiences a decreased or absent ability to use or understand language in human interaction (NANDA).

■ Defining characteristics

Major	*Minor*
Speaks or verbalizes with difficulty	Absence of audible speech
Unable to speak dominant language	Medical regimen/disease process
Difficulty expressing thoughts verbally	interfering with ability to make
Does not or cannot speak	audible sounds (e.g., CVA, ET
Difficulty forming words or	tube, trach)
sentences	Sign language as primary mode of
	communication
	Anatomic defect
	Hearing deficit

■ Suggested alternative diagnoses

Sensory/Perceptual Alterations: Visual, Auditory, Kinesthetic, Gustatory, Tactile, Olfactory (specify)	Thought Processes, Altered Tissue Perfusion, Altered: Cerebral

■ Patient outcomes

Patient communicates needs to staff with minimal frustration.
Patient demonstrates increasing ability to express needs to staff and family.
Patient demonstrates understanding of need to change method of communication to express needs to staff and family.
Patient demonstrates increasing understanding of spoken words and gestures.
Patient communicates satisfaction with alternative means of communication.
Other outcomes specific to patient (specify).

■ Target date

Specify estimated date of completion.

■ Documentation interval

Specify frequency.

■ Nursing interventions

Assess and document patient's communication pattern to facilitate optimal two-way communication.

Assess and document patient's ability to speak, hear, write, read, and understand to establish communication between staff and patient, family and patient.

Explain to patient why he or she cannot speak.

Identify and document patient's primary language.

Use family/significant person or hospital translator, as appropriate. Specify name, phone number, and relationship.

Encourage patient's self-expression in any manner that provides information to staff/family to ensure that patient's needs are being met.

Use flash cards, pad/pencil, gestures, pictures, foreign language vocabulary lists, and the like to facilitate optimal two-way communication.

Encourage patient to communicate slowly and to repeat requests.

Reassure patient that frustration and anger are acceptable and expected.

Encourage frequent family visits to provide stimulation for communication.

Involve the patient and family in development of communication plan. Communication plan is ___.

Speak slowly, distinctly, and quietly, facing the patient.

Provide care in a relaxed, unhurried, nonjudgmental manner.

Provide continuity in nursing assignment to establish trust and reduce frustration.

Consult with physician regarding need for speech therapy, if appropriate.

Encourage patient's communication with staff and family by giving frequent positive reinforcement to patient.

Encourage attendance at group meetings for interpersonal contact. Specify group ___.

Establish one-to-one contact with patient q ___.

Assess and document patient's response to touch, spatial distance, and male/female roles that may influence communication.

Give clear and simple directions, which will avoid overwhelming choices that may add to the patient's confusion. For example, take patient by the arm, saying, "Walk with me now."

Other interventions specific to patient (specify).

Constipation

Related factors: Decreased motility (secondary to aging, Multiple sclerosis, Hirschsprung's disease, and so on), Decreased activity, Decreased fluid intake, Dietary changes, Medications (specify), Painful defecation, Others specific to patient (specify).

Definition: A state in which an individual experiences a change in normal bowel habits characterized by a decrease in frequency and/or passage of hard, dry stools (NANDA).

■ Defining characteristics

Major	*Minor*
Decreased activity level	Abdominal pain
Decreased frequency of defecation	Appetite impairment
Hard, forced stools	Back pain
Palpable mass	Headache
Reported feeling of pressure in rectum	Interference with daily living
Reported feeling of rectal fullness	Use of laxatives
Straining at stool	

■ Suggested alternative diagnoses

Constipation, Colonic
Constipation, Perceived

■ Patient outcomes

Patient reports presence of optimal bowel pattern.
Patient passes stool of usual consistency for patient.
Patient describes dietary requirements necessary to maintain usual bowel pattern.
Patient reports the passage of stool with a reduction of pain and straining.
Patient demonstrates knowledge of bowel regimen necessary to overcome the side-effects of medications.
Other outcomes specific to patient (specify).

■ Target date	■ Documentation interval
Specify estimated date of completion.	Specify frequency.

■ Nursing interventions

Assess and document presence or absence of bowel sounds and abdominal distention in all four quadrants q ___.

Document the passage of flatus.

Assess and document presence of impaction q ___.

Gather baseline data on bowel regimen, activity, and medications. Document patient's usual pattern.

Encourage patient to request pain medication prior to defecation to facilitate painless passage of stool.

Document the color and consistency of first stool postoperatively.

Ask patient and document status regarding frequency, color, and consistency of stool q ___.

Encourage optimal activity to stimulate patient's bowel elimination.

Provide fluids of patient's choice (specify) ____.

Consult with dietitian for increase in fiber in diet.

Request a physician's order for elimination aids, such as dietary bran, stool softeners, and laxatives.

Stress the avoidance of straining during defecation to prevent change in vital signs, dizziness, or bleeding.

Provide privacy and safety for patient during bowel elimination.

Provide care in an accepting, nonjudgmental manner.

Inform patient of possibility of medication-induced constipation.

Instruct patient in bowel elimination aids that will promote optimal bowel pattern at home.

Instruct patient in consequences of long-term laxative use.

Other interventions specific to patient (specify).

Constipation, Colonic

Related factors: Decreased activity, Decreased fluid intake, Less than adequate amounts of fiber and bulk-forming foods in diet, Immobility, Chronic use of medication and enemas, Emotional disturbances, Metabolic conditions such as hypothyroidism, hypokalemia, Fear of moving bowels in hospital environment, Lack of privacy, Change in daily routine, Others specific to patient (specify).

Definition: The state in which an individual's pattern of elimination is characterized by hard, dry stool, which results from delay of passage of food residue (NANDA).

■ **Defining characteristics**

Major	*Minor*
Palpable mass	Abdominal pain
Distended abdomen	Headache
Hard, dry stool	Appetite impairment
Straining at stool	
Decreased frequency of defecation	
Painful defecation	

■ **Suggested alternative diagnoses**

Constipation
Constipation, Perceived

■ **Patient outcomes**

Patient reports presence of optimal bowel pattern.
Patient passes stool of usual consistency and frequency for patient.
Patient describes dietary requirements necessary to maintain usual bowel pattern.
Patient reports the passage of stool with a reduction of pain and straining.
Patient demonstrates knowledge of bowel regimen necessary to overcome the side-effects of medications.
Other outcomes specific to patient (specify).

■ **Target date**	■ **Documentation interval**
Specify estimated date of completion.	Specify frequency.

■ Nursing interventions

Assess and document presence or absence of bowel sounds and abdominal distention in all four quadrants q ___.

Document the passage of flatus.

Assess and document presence of impaction q ___.

Gather baseline data on bowel regimen, activity, and medications. Document patient's usual pattern.

Encourage patient to request pain medication prior to defecation to facilitate painless passage of stool.

Ask patient and document status regarding frequency, color, and consistency of stool q ___.

Encourage optimal activity to stimulate patient's bowel elimination.

Provide fluids of patient's choice (specify).

Consult with dietitian for increase in fiber and bulk-forming food in patient's diet.

Request a physician's order for elimination aids, such as dietary bran, stool softeners, and laxatives.

Stress the avoidance of straining during defecation to prevent change in vital signs, dizziness, or bleeding.

Provide privacy and safety for patient during bowel elimination.

Provide care in an accepting, nonjudgmental manner.

Inform patient of possibility of medication-induced constipation.

Instruct patient in maintaining high-fiber, bulk-forming foods in diet; increasing physical activity; and increasing fluid intake to promote optimal bowel function at home.

Other interventions specific to patient (specify).

Constipation, Perceived

Related factors: Impaired thought processes, Cultural/family health beliefs, Faulty appraisal of normal bowel function, Others specific to patient (specify).

Definition: A state in which an individual makes a self-diagnosis of constipation and ensures a daily bowel movement through the use of laxatives, enemas, and suppositories (NANDA).

■ Defining characteristics

Expected passage of stool at same time every day
Expectation of daily bowel movement, with resulting overuse of laxatives, enemas, and suppositories

■ Suggested alternative diagnoses

Constipation
Constipation, Colonic
Thought Processes, Altered

■ Patient outcomes

Patient acknowledges dependence on use of laxatives, enemas, and suppositories.
Patient verbalizes understanding of need to decrease use of laxatives, enemas, and suppositories.
Patient describes dietary regimen that will more naturally regulate bowel function.
Other outcomes specific to patient (specify).

■ Target date	■ Documentation interval
Specify estimated date of completion.	Specify frequency.

■ **Nursing interventions**

Assess patient's expectation of normal bowel function.

Discuss with patient/family the patient's perceived need to utilize aids for defecation.

Observe, document, and report requests for laxatives, enemas, and/or suppositories.

Assist patient to identify realistic use of laxatives, enemas, and suppositories.

Explore with patient the need to change diet and fluid intake.

Instruct patient and family in diet, fluid, activity, exercise, and the consequence of overuse of laxatives, enemas, and suppositories.

Provide support to patient when behavior change occurs.

Initiate a multidisciplinary care conference involving the patient/family to encourage positive health-seeking behaviors.

Other interventions specific to patient (specify).

Coping, Defensive

Related factors: Situational crisis (specify), Psychological impairment (specify), Others specific to patient (specify).

Definition: The state in which an individual experiences falsely positive self-evaluation based on a self-protective pattern that defends against underlying perceived threats to positive self-regard (NANDA).

■ **Defining characteristics**

Major	*Minor*
Denial of obvious problems/ weaknesses	Superior attitude toward others
Projection of blame/responsibility	History of difficulty in establishing/ maintaining relationships
Rationalization of failures	Hostile laughter or ridicule of others
Grandiosity	Difficulty in reality testing perceptions
Hypersensitivity to slight or criticism	Lack of follow-through or participation in treatment or therapy

■ **Suggested alternative diagnoses**

Coping, Ineffective Individual
Powerlessness
Self-Esteem, Low: Chronic
Self-Esteem, Low: Situational
Thought Processes, Altered

■ **Patient outcomes**

Patient demonstrates decrease in defensiveness.
Patient participates in treatment program.
Patient acknowledges specific problems/conflicts that interfere with social interactions/ relationships.
Other interventions specific to patient (specify).

■ **Target date**

Specify estimated date of completion.

■ **Documentation interval**

Specify frequency.

■ Nursing interventions

Assess degree of defensiveness/denial that interferes with self-assessment.

Identify and discuss the subjects, situations, and people that trigger negative coping behaviors.

Assist patient in recognizing negative coping behaviors.

Teach patient alternative behaviors to obtain positive regard through group therapy, individual therapy, role-playing, and role modeling.

Provide feedback in a supportive environment on how behavior is being perceived by others.

Provide reality testing during times of grandiose behavior, denial of obvious problems, and projected blame/responsibility.

Include family in treatment as needed.

Refer to appropriate community resources.

Other interventions specific to patient (specify).

Coping, Family: Potential for Growth

Related factors: Sufficient achievement of patient's basic health care needs, enabling goals of self-actualization to surface; Others specific to patient (specify).

Definition: A state in which a family member(s) has effectively adapted to patient's health challenge and now exhibits desire and readiness for enhanced growth in regard to self and in relation to the patient (adapted from NANDA).

■ Defining characteristics

Family member begins to recognize growth potential of crisis in relation to own goals, priorities, or relationships
Family member requests information about support groups
Family member verbalizes need to enhance quality of life
Family member promotes and evaluates care for patient

■ Suggested alternative diagnoses

None

■ Family outcomes

Family member(s) identifies and prioritizes personal goals.
Family member(s) develops a plan for personal growth.
Family member(s) implements plan.
Family member(s) evaluates and changes plan as needed.
Other outcomes specific to family (specify).

■ Target date	■ Documentation interval
Specify estimated date of completion.	Specify frequency.

■ Nursing interventions

Provide an opportunity for family member(s) to reflect on impact of patient's illness on family structure and dynamics.

Encourage family member(s) to compare initial response to the crisis with current situation and to recognize change.

Assist family member(s) in identifying and prioritizing personal goals.

Assist family member(s) in developing a plan for personal growth. Plan may include investigation of employment opportunities, school, support groups, enrichment activities, and exercise.

Provide emotional support and availability to family member(s) during implementation, evaluation, and revision of plan.

Other interventions specific to family (specify).

Coping, Ineffective Family: Compromised

Related factors: Inadequate or incorrect information or understanding by family member/close friend, Temporary preoccupation of family member/close friend with own emotional conflicts and personal suffering, Temporary family disorganization and role changes, Situational crisis (specify), Developmental crisis (specify), Patient's diminished support of family member/close friend, Chronic illness or disability, Economic problems, Unrealistic expectations/demands, Lack of mutual decision-making skills, Shift in family's normal power structure, Others specific to patient (specify).

Definition: A state in which a usually supportive family member/close friend provides ineffective comfort/support that may be needed by the patient to manage or master adaptive tasks related to his/her health challenge (adapted from NANDA).

■ Defining characteristics

Patient expresses concern/complaint regarding family members' response
Family member overassists patient
Family member underreacts—e.g., withdraws, ignores, minimizes, refuses to assist
Family member interferes with necessary medical/nursing interventions
Family members are divisive and form unsupportive coalitions
Family verbal interaction with patient is absent or decreased
Family expresses a lack of knowledge
Family attempts to assist with patient care but is unsuccessful
Family is preoccupied with own stressors/conflicts/crises
Family displays emotional lability
Family displays rigid role boundaries

■ Suggested alternative diagnoses

Caregiver Role Strain (Actual/High Risk)
Coping, Ineffective Family: Disabling
Family Processes, Altered
Parental Role Conflict

■ Family outcomes

Family identifies conflicting coping styles.
Family expresses unresolved feelings.
Family acknowledges needs of patient.
Family acknowledges needs of family unit.
Family uses more flexible problem-solving strategies.
Family begins to demonstrate effective interpersonal skills.
Family participates in developing and implementing a treatment plan.
Family expresses increased ability to cope with changes in family structure and dynamics.
Other outcomes specific to patient (specify).

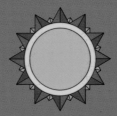

1992 NANDA Approved Nursing Diagnostic Categories

Activity Intolerance
Activity Intolerance: High Risk
Adjustment, Impaired
Airway Clearance, Ineffective
Anxiety
Aspiration: High Risk
Body Image Disturbance
Body Temperature, Altered: High Risk
Bowel Incontinence
Breast-Feeding, Effective (Potential for Enhanced)
Breast-Feeding, Ineffective
Breast-Feeding, Interrupted[1]
Breathing Pattern, Ineffective
Cardiac Output, Decreased
Caregiver Role Strain (Actual/High Risk)[1]
Communication, Impaired: Verbal
Constipation
Constipation, Colonic
Constipation, Perceived
Coping, Defensive
Coping, Family: Potential for Growth
Coping, Ineffective Family: Compromised
Coping, Ineffective Family: Disabling
Coping, Ineffective Individual
Decisional Conflict (specify)
Denial, Ineffective
Diarrhea
Disuse Syndrome: High Risk
Diversional Activity Deficit

Dysfunctional Ventilatory Weaning Response (DVWR)[1]
Dysreflexia
Family Processes, Altered
Fatigue
Fear
Fluid Volume Deficit
Fluid Volume Deficit: High Risk
Fluid Volume Excess
Gas Exchange, Impaired
Grieving, Anticipatory
Grieving, Dysfunctional
Growth and Development, Altered
Health Maintenance, Altered
Health-Seeking Behaviors (specify)
Home Maintenance Management, Impaired
Hopelessness
Hyperthermia
Hypothermia
Infant Feeding Pattern, Ineffective[1]
Infection: High Risk
Injury: High Risk
Knowledge Deficit (specify)
Mobility, Impaired Physical
Noncompliance (specify)
Nutrition, Altered: Less Than Body Requirements
Nutrition, Altered: More Than Body Requirements

Continued

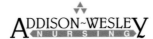

ADDISON~WESLEY
NURSING
A DIVISION OF
THE BENJAMIN/CUMMINGS PUBLISHING COMPANY, INC.

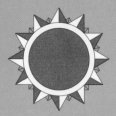

Nutrition, Altered: High Risk for More Than Body Requirements
Oral Mucous Membrane, Altered
Pain [Acute]
Pain, Chronic
Parental Role Conflict
Parenting, Altered
Parenting, Altered: High Risk
Peripheral Neurovascular Dysfunction: High Risk[1]
Personal Identity Disturbance
Poisoning: High Risk
Post-Trauma Response
Powerlessness
Protection, Altered
Rape-Trauma Syndrome
Rape-Trauma Syndrome: Compound Reaction
Rape-Trauma Syndrome: Silent Reaction
Relocation Stress Syndrome
Role Performance, Altered
Self-Care Deficit: Bathing/Hygiene
Self-Care Deficit: Dressing/Grooming
Self-Care Deficit: Feeding
Self-Care Deficit: Toileting
Self-Esteem Disturbance
Self-Esteem, Low: Chronic
Self-Esteem, Low: Situational
Self-Mutilation: High Risk
Sensory/Perceptual Alterations: Visual, Auditory, Kinesthetic, Gustatory, Tactile, Olfactory (specify)
Sexual Dysfunction

Sexuality Patterns, Altered
Skin Integrity, Impaired
Skin Integrity, Impaired: High Risk
Sleep Pattern Disturbance
Social Interaction, Impaired
Social Isolation
Spiritual Distress
Spontaneous Ventilation, Inability to Sustain[1]
Suffocation: High Risk
Swallowing, Impaired
Therapeutic Regimen Management, Ineffective Individual[1]
Thermoregulation, Impaired
Thought Processes, Altered
Tissue Integrity, Impaired
Tissue Perfusion, Altered: Renal, Cerebral, Cardiopulmonary, Gastrointestinal, Peripheral (specify type)
Trauma: High Risk
Unilateral Neglect
Urinary Elimination, Altered
Urinary Incontinence, Functional
Urinary Incontinence, Reflex
Urinary Incontinence, Stress
Urinary Incontinence, Total
Urinary Incontinence, Urge
Urinary Retention
Violence, High Risk: Self-Directed or Directed at Others

[1]*Diagnoses accepted in 1992*

■ **Target date** ■ **Documentation interval**

Specify estimated date of completion. Specify frequency.

■ **Nursing interventions**

Assess interaction between patient and family, being alert for potential destructive behaviors.
Assist family in identifying personal strengths.
Provide information about specific health challenge and necessary coping skills.
Discuss the common responses to health challenges, e.g., anxiety, dependency, depression.
Encourage family to verbalize feelings.
Discuss with family effective ways to demonstrate feelings.
Assist family in realistically identifying the needs of patient and family unit.
Promote an open, trusting relationship with family.
Explore impact of conflicting coping styles on family relationships.
Assist family in identifying behaviors that may be hindering prescribed treatment.
Encourage family to recognize changes in interpersonal relationships.
Encourage family to identify needed role changes to maintain family integrity.
Teach, role model, and reinforce communication skills, which may include active listening, reflection, "I" statements, conflict resolution.
Assist family with decision-making and problem-solving skills.
Assist family members in assuming new roles.
Provide structure to family interaction. Consider:
    Which family member(s) will visit, based on patient's treatment plan.
    Length of visiting time.
    Content of interaction.
    Staff support during visit.
Encourage family to visit patient whenever possible. Provide privacy to facilitate family interactions.
Teach the family those skills required for care of patient. Specify.
Encourage family to participate in patient's care.
Initiate a multidisciplinary patient care conference, involving the patient/family in problem solving and facilitation of communication.
Provide continuity of care by maintaining effective communication between staff members through nurse report, patient care conferences, and care planning.
Encourage family to express concerns to help plan posthospital care.
Explore available hospital and community resources with family.
Refer family members to appropriate support systems to encourage attention to needs of self.
Request social service consultation to help the family determine posthospitalization needs and identify sources of community support.
Other interventions specific to family (specify).

Coping, Ineffective Family: Disabling

Related factors: Chronically unresolved feelings (specify guilt, anxiety, hostility, despair, and so on), Highly ambivalent family relationships, Substance-abusing family member, Emotionally disturbed family member, Use of violence to manage conflict, Child sexual/physical abuse, Others specific to family (specify).

Definition: Behavior of a significant family member that disables his/her own capacity, as well as the patient's capacity to perform effectively tasks essential to either person's adaptation to the health challenge (adapted from NANDA).

■ Defining characteristics

Neglectful care of patient in regard to basic human needs and/or illness treatment
Distortion of reality of patient's health problem, including extreme denial about its existence or severity
Rejection of patient
Intolerance
Psychosomatic symptoms
Family member displaying illness signs of patient
Agitation
Abandonment
Desertion
Depression
Aggression/hostility
Neglectful relationships with other family members
Patient displaying helpless, inactive dependence
Disregarding patient's needs
Decisions and actions by family that are detrimental to economic or social well-being
Impaired restructuring of a meaningful life for self
Impaired individualization
Inability to make decisions and solve problems

■ Suggested alternative diagnoses

Caregiver Role Strain (Actual/High Risk)
Coping, Ineffective Family: Compromised
Coping, Ineffective Individual
Parenting, Altered
Violence, High Risk: Self-Directed or Directed at Others

■ **Family outcomes**

Family identifies conflicting coping styles.
Family expresses unresolved feelings.
Family acknowledges needs of patient.
Family acknowledges needs of family unit.
Family begins to demonstrate effective interpersonal skills.
Family demonstrates ability to resolve conflict without use of violence.
Family participates in effective problem solving.
Family participates in treatment plan.
Family identifies and maintains intrafamily sexual boundaries.
Other outcomes specific to family (specify).

■ **Target date**	■ **Documentation interval**
Specify estimated date of completion.	Specify frequency.

■ **Nursing interventions**

Assess interaction between patient and family, being alert for potential destructive behaviors.
Assist family in recognizing the problem, e.g., managing conflict with violence, sexual abuse.
Report indications of physical/sexual abuse as directed by law to appropriate authorities.
Discuss with family effective ways to demonstrate feelings.
Assist family in realistically identifying the needs of patient and family unit.
Explore impact of conflicting coping styles on family relationships.
Teach, role model, and reinforce communications skills, which may include active listening, reflection, "I" statements, conflict resolution, and nonviolent methods of expressing anger.
Discuss how violence is a learned behavior and can be transmitted to offspring.
Provide structure to family interaction. Consider:
    Which family member(s) will visit, based on patient's treatment plan.
    Length of visiting time.
    Content of interaction.
    Staff support during visit.
Teach the family those skills required for care of patient. Specify.
Initiate a multidisciplinary patient care conference, involving the patient/family in problem solving and facilitation of communication.
Provide continuity of care by maintaining effective communication between staff members through nurse report, patient care conferences, and care planning.
Encourage family participation in all group meetings.
Encourage family to express concerns and to help plan posthospital care.
Refer family/individual members to support groups, psychiatric treatment, social services (e.g., chemical dependence programs, Parents United, Incest Survivors Anonymous, child protective services, battered wives' shelters).
Other interventions specific to patient (specify).

Coping, Ineffective Individual

Related factors: Personal vulnerability in a maturational crisis (specify), Personal vulnerability in a situational crisis (specify), Others specific to patient (specify).

Definition: A state in which an individual is unable to problem-solve or use adaptive behaviors to meet life's demands and roles (NANDA).

■ **Defining characteristics**

Verbalization of inability to cope or inability to ask for help[1]
Inability to problem-solve[1]
Destructive behavior toward self and others
Change in usual communication patterns
Expressing unrealistic expectations
Reported substance abuse
Inability to meet role expectations
High illness rate
Verbal manipulation
Inability to meet basic needs
Inappropriate use of defense mechanisms
High rate of accidents
Evidence of physical/psychologic abuse
Alteration in societal participation

■ **Suggested alternative diagnoses**

Anxiety
Fear
Grieving, Dysfunctional
Hopelessness
Post-Trauma Response
Powerlessness
Rape-Trauma Syndrome: Compound Reaction
Rape-Trauma Syndrome: Silent Reaction
Self-Esteem, Low: Chronic
Self-Esteem, Low: Situational
Self-Mutilation: High Risk
Violence, High Risk: Self-Directed or Directed at Others

■ **Patient outcomes**

Patient's verbal and nonverbal expressions are applicable to situation.
Patient identifies personal strengths that may promote effective coping.
Patient initiates conversation.
Patient participates in activities of daily living.
Patient demonstrates interest in diversional activities.
Patient participates in decision-making process.
Patient verbalizes plan for either accepting or changing the situation.
Other outcomes specific to patient (specify).

■ **Target date**	■ **Documentation interval**
Specify estimated date of completion.	Specify frequency.

■ **Nursing interventions**

Assess potential for self-destructive behaviors, and document.
Assess aggressive behaviors.
Encourage patient to demonstrate feelings.
Encourage patient to request family visitation whenever possible.
Encourage patient to initiate conversations with others.
Assist patient in identifying personal strengths.
Encourage patient to express concerns and help solve problems.
Encourage patient involvement in planning care activities.
Encourage patient to participate in activity.
Promote a trusting relationship with patient and family.
Involve hospital resources in provision of emotional support for patient and family.
Initiate a patient care conference to review patient's coping mechanisms and to establish a plan of care.
Assist patient in developing a plan for accepting or changing situation.
Other interventions specific to patient (specify).

---

[1]Must be present to justify diagnosis.

Decisional Conflict (specify)

Related factors: Perceived threat to value system, Lack of experience with decision making, Interference with decision making, Lack of relevant information, Multiple or divergent sources of information, Lack of support system, Interference with support system, Unclear personal values/beliefs, Others specific to patient (specify).

Definition: State of uncertainty about course of action to be taken when choice among competing actions involves risk, loss, or challenge to personal life values (NANDA).

■ **Defining characteristics**

Major	*Minor*
Verbalizing undesired consequences of alternative actions being considered	Displaying signs of distress or tension (e.g., increased heart rate, restlessness, increased muscle tension)
Verbalizing uncertainty about choices	Focusing on self
Vacillating between alternative choices	Questioning personal values and beliefs while attempting a decision
Delaying decision making	Verbalizing feeling of distress while attempting a decision

■ **Suggested alternative diagnoses**

Parental Role Conflict
Therapeutic Regimen Management, Ineffective Individual

■ **Patient outcomes**

Patient acknowledges the advantages/disadvantages of available choices.
Patient evaluates available choices in relation to personal values.
Patient decides on course of action.
Patient reports a decrease in tension or distress.
Other outcomes specific to patient (specify).

■ **Target date**	■ **Documentation interval**
Specify estimated date of completion.	Specify frequency.

■ **Nursing interventions**

Assess patient's understanding of available choices.

Provide accurate information about choices.

Explore with patient the advantages and disadvantages of each choice.

Help patient decide the importance of each advantage and disadvantage through discussion, "weighing," prioritizing, and eliminating obviously unacceptable choices.

Assist patient in identifying a course of action and adapt as necessary.

Encourage patient to discuss decision and process with the health care team, family, and significant others.

Evaluate patient's level of tension or distress.

Use resources as appropriate.

Other interventions specific to patient (specify).

Denial, Ineffective

Related factor: Specific to patient.

Definition: The state of a conscious or unconscious attempt to disavow the knowledge or meaning of an event to reduce anxiety/fear to the detriment of health (NANDA).

■ **Defining characteristics**

Major

Delay in seeking or refusal of health care attention to the detriment to health
Failure to perceive personal relevance of symptoms or danger

Minor

Minimizing symptoms
Displacing source of symptoms to other organs
Inappropriate affect
Failure to admit fear of death or invalidism
Inability to admit impact of disease in life pattern
Displacing fear of impact of the condition
Making dismissive gestures or comments when speaking of distressing events

■ **Suggested alternative diagnoses**

Coping, Defensive
Coping, Ineffective Family: Compromised
Coping, Ineffective Family: Disabling
Coping, Ineffective Individual
Grieving, Dysfunctional
Noncompliance (specify)
Rape-Trauma Syndrome: Silent Reaction
Therapeutic Regimen Management, Ineffective Individual

■ **Patient outcomes**

Patient begins to acknowledge symptoms.
Patient recognizes significance of symptoms.
Patient reports significant symptoms.
Other outcomes specific to patient (specify).

■ **Target date**

Specify estimated date of completion.

■ **Documentation interval**

Specify frequency.

■ **Nursing interventions**

Assess patient's understanding of symptoms/illness.
Establish a therapeutic relationship with patient that will allow exploration of denial.
Engage patient in discussion about anxiety, fears, symptoms, and impact of illness.
Include patient/family in a multidisciplinary conference to develop a plan of action.
> Plan may include:
> Teaching recognition of symptoms and desired patient response.
> Using every opportunity to reinforce consequences of patient's actions.
> Meeting with patients in similar situations to learn new ways to cope and to decrease anxiety and fear.
> Arranging for follow-up/support after discharge.

Other interventions specific to patient (specify).

Diarrhea

Related factors: Dietary changes, Increased intestinal motility secondary to ___, Excessive alcohol intake, Impaction, Medications (specify), Stress, Food intolerance, Others specific to patient (specify).

Definition: A state in which an individual experiences a change in normal bowel habits characterized by the frequent passage of loose, fluid, unformed stools (NANDA).

■ Defining characteristics

Major	*Minor*
Abdominal cramping	Change in color of stool
Abdominal pain	
Urgency to defecate	
Change in usual consistency, frequency, and volume of stool	
Loose/liquid stool	

■ Suggested alternative diagnosis

Bowel Incontinence

■ Patient outcomes

Patient reports presence of optimal bowel pattern.
Patient passes stool of usual consistency.
Patient passes stool with decreasing frequency.
Patient describes dietary requirements to maintain usual bowel pattern.
Patient has weight gain.
Patient's hygiene is adequate to prevent skin breakdown.
Other outcomes specific to patient (specify).

■ Target date   ■ Documentation interval

Specify estimated date of completion.   Specify frequency.

■ **Nursing interventions**

Assess and document frequency, color, and consistency of stool q ___.

Assess and document impaction q ___.

Assess and document condition of perianal skin q ___.

Monitor laboratory values (electrolytes, CBC), and report abnormalities.

Assess and document skin turgor and condition of oral mucosa as indicators of dehydration q ___.

Weigh patient daily.

Guaiac stools q ___.

Have patient identify usual bowel pattern. Document.

Encourage patient to identify stressors that may contribute to diarrhea. Document.

Request order from physician for antidiarrheal, antispasmodic, and/or topical medications.

Inform patient of possibility of medication-induced diarrhea.

Provide care in an accepting, nonjudgmental manner.

Provide fluids of patient's choice (specify) ___.

Consult with dietitian for adjustment of dietary fiber.

Consult with pediatrician for alternative type of feeding.

Provide privacy and safety for patient during bowel elimination.

Instruct patient in diet and use of antidiarrheal medications to promote optimal bowel pattern at home.

Other interventions specific to patient (specify).

Disuse Syndrome: High Risk

Risk factors: Paralysis, Mechanical immobilization, Prescribed immobilization, Severe pain, Altered level of consciousness, Others specific to patient (specify).

Definition: A state in which an individual is at risk for deterioration of body systems as the result of prescribed or unavoidable inactivity (NANDA).

The authors have chosen to modify the format of this nursing care plan to reflect the complexity and diversity of the disuse syndrome. The outcomes and interventions selected are determined by the patient's affected body system and the degree of disuse. For specific patient outcomes and nursing interventions, see these suggested nursing diagnoses:

Activity Intolerance: High Risk

Bowel Incontinence

Breathing Pattern, Ineffective

Caregiver Role Strain (Actual/High Risk)

Constipation

Coping, Ineffective Family: Disabling

Coping, Ineffective Individual

Denial, Ineffective

Infection: High Risk

Injury: High Risk

Mobility, Impaired Physical

Nutrition, Altered: Less Than Body Requirements

Peripheral Neurovascular Dysfunction: High Risk

Powerlessness

Self-Care Deficit: Bathing/Hygiene, Dressing/Grooming, Feeding,
    Toileting (specify)

Sensory/Perceptual Alterations: All (specify)

Sexuality Patterns, Altered

Skin Integrity, Impaired: High Risk

Sleep Pattern Disturbance

Swallowing, Impaired

Tissue Perfusion, Altered: Peripheral

Urinary Incontinence, Reflex

Urinary Incontinence, Total

Urinary Retention

Diversional Activity Deficit

Related factors: Deficit in social skills, Disturbance in motivation, Impaired perception of reality, Frequent/lengthy medical treatments, Forced inactivity, Prolonged bed rest, Long-term hospitalization, Others specific to patient (specify).

Definition: The state in which an individual experiences decreased stimulation from or decreased interest/engagement in recreational leisure activities (NANDA).

■ Defining characteristics

Expressing apathy, boredom
Complaining of inability to initiate or continue with usual activity
Anger, hostility
Flat affect
Increase in daytime sleep periods
Restlessness
Disruptive behavior
Withdrawn behavior

■ Suggested alternative diagnoses

Adjustment, Impaired
Social Interaction, Impaired

■ Patient outcomes

Patient verbalizes acceptance of limitations that interfere with usual leisure activities.
Patient helps identify activity alternatives that may provide stimulation.
Patient demonstrates socially acceptable behaviors during activities.
Other outcomes specific to patient (specify).

■ Target date   ■ Documentation interval

Specify estimated date of completion.   Specify frequency.

■ **Nursing interventions**

Encourage patient to verbalize feelings and concerns regarding limitations.

Provide appropriate stimuli, such as music, games, visitors, and relaxation therapy, to vary monotonous routines and stimulate thought.

Alternate patient care routines, involving patient in plans.

Identify resources, such as volunteers and occupational therapists, that could assist patient in recreational/leisure activities.

Provide compatible roommate, if possible.

Introduce patient to other patients who have successfully dealt with similar situations.

Encourage family, friends, and significant persons to visit.

Encourage patient to participate in activities of interest that can be provided during hospitalization. Specify ___.

Introduce and encourage new or alternative leisure-time activities. Specify.

Other interventions specific to patient (specify).

Dysfunctional Ventilatory Weaning Response (DVWR)

Related factors: *Physical:* Ineffective airway clearance, Sleep pattern disturbance, Inadequate nutrition, Uncontrolled pain or discomfort; *Psychological:* Knowledge deficit of the weaning process, Patient role, Patient perceived inefficacy about the ability to wean, Decreased motivation, Decreased self-esteem, Anxiety: moderate, severe, Fear, Hopelessness, Powerlessness, Insufficient trust in the nurse; *Situational:* Uncontrolled episodic energy demands or problems, Inappropriate pacing of diminished ventilator support, Inadequate social support, Adverse environment (noisy, active environment, negative events in the room, low nurse-patient ratio, extended nurse absence from bedside, unfamiliar nursing staff), History of ventilator dependence > 1 week, History of multiple unsuccessful weaning attempts.

Definition: A state in which a patient cannot adjust to lowered levels of mechanical ventilator support, which interrupts and prolongs the weaning process (NANDA).

■ Defining characteristics

Mild DVWR

Major	*Minor*
Restlessness	Responds to lowered levels of mechanical ventilator support with:
Slight increased respiratory rate from baseline	Expressed feelings of increased need for oxygen, breathing discomfort, fatigue, warmth
	Queries about possible machine malfunction
	Increased concentration on breathing

Moderate DVWR

Major	*Minor*
Responds to lowered levels of mechanical ventilator support with:	Hypervigilance to activities
Slight increase from baseline blood pressure < 20mm Hg	Inability to respond to coaching
Slight increase from baseline heart rate < 20 beats/minute	Inability to cooperate
Baseline increase in respiratory rate < 5 breaths/minute	Apprehension
	Diaphoresis
	Eye widening ("wide-eyed" look)
	Decreased air entry on auscultation
	Color changes; pale, slight cyanosis
	Slight respiratory accessory muscle use

Severe DVWR

Major

Responds to lowered levels of mechanical ventilatory support with:
Agitation
Deterioration in arterial blood gases from current baseline
Increase from baseline blood pressure >20 mm Hg
Increase from baseline heart rate >20 beats/minute
Respiratory rate increases significantly from baseline

Minor

Profuse diaphoresis
Full respiratory accessory muscle use
Shallow, gasping breaths
Paradoxical abdominal breathing
Discoordinated breathing with the ventilator
Decreased level of consciousness
Adventitious breath sounds, audible airway secretions
Cyanosis

■ **Suggested alternative diagnosis**

Gas Exchange, Impaired

■ **Patient outcomes**

Patient is physiologically stable for weaning process.
Patient is psychologically and emotionally ready for weaning process.
Patient demonstrates understanding of the weaning process and his/her role in achieving weaning process goals.
Patient participates in goal setting for weaning process.
Patient demonstrates necessary physical and emotional resources to achieve weaning goals.
Patient achieves established weaning goals.
Other outcomes specific to patient (specify).

■ **Target date**

Specify estimated date of completion.

■ **Documentation interval**

Specify frequency.

■ **Nursing interventions**

Assess patient's readiness to wean by considering the following respiratory indicators:
   Arterial blood gases stable with $PaO_2 > 60$ on 40–60% oxygen.
   Vital capacity > 13 ml/kg ideal body weight.
   Length of time on ventilator.
   Maximum inspiratory force > –25 cm H_2O (normal –80 to –1000) so independent respiration can be initiated.
   Unassisted tidal volume > 5 ml/kg ideal body weight.
   Cough effectively enough to handle secretions.
   Stable spontaneous respiratory rate < 35 breaths/minute (BPM).
Assess patient's readiness to wean by considering the following non-respiratory indicators:
   Stable heart rate and rhythm.
   Electrolytes within normal limits for patient.
   Hemoglobin and hematocrit within normal limits for patient.
   Adequate nutritional status as evidenced by acceptable serum
      albumin, transferrin, midarm muscle circumference > 15 percentile.
   Tolerable pain or discomfort level.
   Absence of fever and/or infection.
   Normal blood pressure for patient.
   Adequate rest and sleep.
   Improving body strength and endurance.
   Psychological/emotional readiness.
   Absence of constipation, diarrhea, or ileus.
Establish effective methods of communication between patient and others (e.g., writing, blinking eyes, squeezing hand, etc.).
Monitor patient's response to current medications and correlate with weaning goals.
Discuss weaning process and goals with physician and respiratory care practitioner, including patient's present and pre-existing medical condition(s).
Establish a trusting relationship that instills patient's confidence in nurse to assist patient with weaning process.
Instruct patient/family in weaning process and goals, which should include:
   Why weaning is necessary.
   How patient may feel as process evolves.
   Participation required by patient.
   What patient can expect from nurse.
   Participation of family.
Encourage self-care to increase sense of control and participation in own care.
   Normalize ADLs to patient's tolerance.
Initiate weaning process by:
   Understanding the rationale for weaning orders [use of CPAP (Continuous Positive Airway Pressure); SIMV (Synchronized Intermittent Mandatory Ventilation); PSV (Pressure Support Ventilation); MMV (Mandatory Minute Ventilation)]; or T-piece.
   Explain procedure to patient and family.

Check equipment to make sure it is attached to oxygen.

Check tubing for kinks and excessive moisture.

Check that settings are as ordered.

Check for presence of bilateral breath sounds.

Measure and record baseline respiratory rate, heart rate, blood pressure, EKG rhythm, lung sounds, vital capacity, tidal volume, inspiratory force, saturated oxygen via pulse oxymeter.

Preoxygenate, hyperinflate, suction, reoxygenate patient prior to weaning.

Stay with patient during weaning time to provide coaching and reassurance.

Provide a quiet environment during weaning time.

Provide diversions such as television or radio.

Sit patient in an upright position to decrease abdominal pressure on the diaphragm allowing for better lung expansion.

Start the weaning time when patient has rested and is awake and alert.

Check vital signs and patient for indicators of non-tolerance or fatigue q5–15 minutes. Reconnect patient to ventilator at pre-weaning settings if indicators of non-tolerance occur.

Document weaning process and patient's tolerance in nurses notes or flow sheet.

Document in nursing care plan those strategies that promote success with weaning process to ensure consistency (e.g., communication method with patient, family participation, coaching methods, etc.).

Reevaluate appropriateness of weaning process with physician if weaning goals are not attainable.

Other interventions specific to patient (specify).

Dysreflexia

Related factors: Bladder distention in spinal cord injury, Bowel distention in spinal cord injury, Skin irritation or skin lesion in spinal cord injury.

Definition: The state in which an individual with a spinal cord injury at T7 or above experiences a life-threatening, uninhibited sympathetic response of the nervous system to a noxious stimulus (NANDA).

■ Defining characteristics

Major	Minor
Bradycardia	Chills
Tachycardia	Blurred vision
Diaphoresis above injury	Nasal congestion
Red splotches on skin	Chest pain
Pallor below injury	Metallic taste in mouth
Paroxysmal hypertension (sudden periodic elevation of blood pressure, where systolic is >140 and diastolic is >90)	Conjunctival congestion
	Goose bumps
	Horner's syndrome (contraction of pupil, partial ptosis of eyelid, enophthalmos, absence of sweating over affected side of face)
Pounding diffuse headache	Paresthesia

■ Suggested alternative diagnosis

Urinary Retention

■ Patient outcomes

Patient identifies early signs and symptoms of dysreflexia.
Patient demonstrates ability to maintain bowel and bladder routine.
Patient's blood pressure maintained at ___ or less.
Other outcomes specific to patient (specify).

■ Target date	■ Documentation interval
Specify estimated date of completion.	Specify frequency.

■ Nursing interventions

Assess patient's knowledge of condition, including history of previous episodes, early signs and symptoms, and bowel and bladder regimen.

Obtain baseline temperature, blood pressure, and pulse. Baseline temperature, blood pressure, and pulse are ___.

Assess for bladder distention q4 hours.

Assess skin condition at least daily, noting any reddened areas above level of spinal cord injury.

Assess for bowel elimination q day.

Instruct patient in early signs and symptoms of condition: pounding headache, flushing diaphoresis of face and thorax.

Ask patient to report presence of any early signs and symptoms of condition.

During onset of crisis, carry out management plan as follows:

Stop activity, and have someone notify physician.

Decrease blood pressure by elevating head of bed or putting patient in sitting position.

Monitor blood pressure q3–5 minutes.

Quickly eliminate noxious stimulus in the following order:

Bladder: Check catheter for patency, or catheterize patient.

Bowel: If distended, apply anesthetic ointment to rectal area, and disimpact. Consider enema or flatus tube.

Body temperature: Maintain normal body temperature.

Administer antihypertensive medications as ordered.

Review with caretaker needed interventions during onset of crisis.

Other interventions specific to patient (specify).

Family Processes, Altered

Related factors: Change in family roles, Change in family structure, Hospitalization/change in environment, Illness/disability of family member, Separation of family members, Lack of adequate support system, Unmet expectations for pregnancy, Unmet expectations for childbirth, Unmet expectations for child, Others specific to family (specify).

Definition: The state in which a family that normally functions effectively experiences dysfunction (NANDA).

■ Defining characteristics

Inability to accept/express wide range of feelings
Absence of family interaction
Entry of new family member into home (e.g., elder, newborn)
Family hindrance of nursing/medical care
Verbal hostility between family members/patient/staff
Poorly communicated family rules, rituals, or symbols
Inability to express/accept feelings of members
Lack of family involvment in community activities
Rigidity in function and roles
Inability to accept/receive help
Inability to deal with traumatic event constructively
Failure to accomplish current developmental tasks
Differing expectations expressed by family members
Inability of family system to meet physical, emotional, and spiritual needs of its members

■ Suggested alternative diagnoses

Caregiver Role Strain (Actual/High Risk)
Coping, Ineffective Family: Compromised
Coping, Ineffective Family: Disabling
Grieving, Dysfunctional
Parental Role Conflict

■ Family outcomes

Family members acknowledge change in family roles.
Family members identify coping patterns.
Family members participate in decision-making processes regarding posthospital care.
Other outcomes specific to family (specify).

■ Target date	■ Documentation interval
Specify estimated date of completion.	Specify frequency.

■ **Nursing interventions**

Assess interaction between patient and family, being alert for potential destructive behaviors.

Encourage family to verbalize feelings.

Discuss with family appropriate ways to demonstrate feelings.

Promote an open, trusting relationship with family.

Encourage family to visit patient whenever possible. Provide privacy to facilitate family interactions.

Assist family in identifying personal strengths.

Assist family in identifying behaviors that may be hindering prescribed treatment.

Encourage family to participate in patient's care.

Provide positive reinforcement for effective use of coping mechanisms.

Provide continuity of care by maintaining effective communication between staff members through nurse report, patient care conferences, and care planning.

Initiate a multidisciplinary patient care conference, involving the patient/family in problem solving and facilitation of communication.

Encourage family to express concerns and to help plan posthospital care.

Teach the family those skills required for care of patient. Specify ___.

Explore available hospital and community resources with family.

Request social service consultation to help the family determine posthospitalization needs and identify sources of community support.

Refer family to a financial counselor.

Other interventions specific to family (specify).

Fatigue

Related factors: Decreased/increased metabolic energy production, states of discomfort, Increased energy requirements to perform activities of daily living, Excessive social and/or role demands, Overwhelming psychologic or emotional demands, Altered body chemistry (e.g., medications, drug withdrawal, chemotherapy), Others specific to patient (specify).

Definition: An overwhelming, sustained sense of exhaustion and decreased capacity for physical and mental work (NANDA).

■ Defining characteristics

Major	*Minor*
Inability to maintain usual routines	Inability to concentrate
Verbalization of unremitting and	Decreased libido
overwhelming lack of energy	Decreased performance
	Increased physical complaints
	Emotional lability
	Lethargy, listlessness
	Disinterest in surroundings
	Irritability
	Accident-proneness

■ Suggested alternative diagnoses

Activity Intolerance
Activity Intolerance: High Risk
Cardiac Output, Decreased
Coping, Ineffective Individual
Pain [Acute]

■ Patient outcomes

Patient demonstrates ability to maintain usual activity level and social interaction.
Patient demonstrates increasing ability to concentrate.
Patient acknowledges disease process/condition that exacerbates symptoms of fatigue.
Patient identifies measures that modify environment to reduce fatigue.
Patient differentiates psychologic from physical factors that may cause fatigue.
Other outcomes specific to patient (specify).

■ Target date   ■ Documentation interval

Specify estimated date of completion.   Specify frequency.

■ **Nursing interventions**

Assess and document patient's level of fatigue q ___.

Encourage patient to report onset of pain that may produce fatigue (severity, location, precipitating factors). Document.

Encourage patient to report activities that increase fatigue.

Encourage patient to identify measures that prevent or modify fatigue.

Plan activities with patient/family that minimize fatigue. Plan may include:

Setting small, realistic, attainable goals for patient that decrease fatigue. Specify goals ___.

Providing rest periods during activities.

Providing positive reinforcement for increase in activity.

Assisting with ADLs as needed. Specify assistance needed.

Including family in plan to minimize fatigue as appropriate. Specify.

Discuss with patient/family ways to modify home environment to maintain usual activity level/social interaction and to minimize fatigue.

Plan activities to allow time for adequate rest, avoid unnecessary procedures during resting period, and limit visitation during resting period.

Instruct patient in the relationship of fatigue to disease process/condition.

Assist patient in identifying measures that increase concentration. Consider:

Completing simple tasks.

Prioritizing necessary tasks.

Initiating tasks after rest periods.

Initiating tasks after pain medication.

Reducing surrounding distractions (noise, people, television).

Other interventions specific to patient (specify).

Fear

Related factors: Environmental stressor/hospitalization, Powerlessness, Real or imagined threat to own well-being, Implications for future pregnancies, Real or imagined threat to child, Others specific to patient (specify).

Definition: Feeling of dread related to an identifiable source which the person validates (NANDA).

■ Defining characteristics

Ability to identify object of fear

■ Suggested alternative diagnoses

Anxiety
Post-Trauma Response
Rape-Trauma Syndrome

■ Patient outcomes

Patient names known sources of fear.
Patient demonstrates behaviors that may reduce fear.
Patient reports reasonable comfort.
Other outcomes specific to patient (specify).

■ Target date

Specify estimated date of completion.

■ Documentation interval

Specify frequency.

■ **Nursing interventions**

Encourage patient to differentiate real from imagined threat to well-being by discussing the sources of fear.

Convey acceptance of the patient's perception of fear to encourage open communication regarding the source of the fear.

Encourage and help patient to express the contributing factors that have produced fear.

Provide frequent verbal and nonverbal reassurances that may assist in reducing the patient's fear state. Avoid clichés.

Remove the source of the patient's fear whenever possible.

Provide patient with information/interaction regarding procedures and hospital routine.

Provide frequent, positive reinforcement when patient demonstrates behaviors that may reduce or eliminate fear.

Encourage a patient/physician discussion of the patient's fear.

Initiate a multidisciplinary patient care conference to develop a plan of care. Specify plan.

Assess need for social service and/or psychiatric intervention.

Provide continuity of patient care through patient assignment and use of care plan.

Other interventions specific to patient (specify).

Fluid Volume Deficit

Related factors: Abnormal blood loss (specify), Excessive continuous consumption of alcohol, Inadequate fluid intake secondary to ___, Failure of regulatory mechanisms (as in diabetes insipidus, hyperaldosteronism), Abnormal fluid loss (specify), Others specific to patient (specify).

Definition: The state in which an individual experiences vascular, cellular, or intracellular dehydration (NANDA).

■ **Defining characteristics**

Major	Minor
Change in urine output	Hypotension
Change in urine concentration	Thirst
Sudden weight loss or gain	Increased pulse rate
Decreased venous filling	Decreased skin turgor
Hemoconcentration	Decreased pulse volume/pressure
Change in serum sodium	Change in mental state
	Increased body temperature
	Dry skin
	Dry mucous membrane
	Weakness

■ **Suggested alternative diagnosis**

Tissue Perfusion, Altered: Renal

■ **Patient outcomes**

Patient is oriented to person, place, and time.
Patient has moist mucous membranes.
Patient's vital signs are within normal limits for patient. Specify normal limits.
Patient's serum electrolytes, hemoglobin, and hematocrit are within normal range for patient. State normal range.
Patient's urine is less concentrated. Specify baseline specific gravity.
Patient reports no thirst.
Patient reports no weakness.
Other outcomes specific to patient (specify).

■ **Target date**

Specify estimated date of completion.

■ **Documentation interval**

Specify frequency.

■ Nursing interventions

Assess and document skin turgor and mucous membranes q ___ as parameters for adequate hydration.

Assess and document specific gravity and color of urine q ___.

Assess and document color, amount, and frequency of emesis, diarrhea, and other drainage.

Assess and document vital signs q ___.

Assess and document orientation to person, place, and time q___.

Assess and document dressing changes to evaluate fluid loss from wounds.

Assess and document skin temperature, dryness, and color.

Assess and document intake and output.

Assess and document for active bleeding. Specify location.

Identify contributing factors that may aggravate dehydration, such as medications, fever, stress, medical orders.

Weigh patient q ___.

Encourage oral fluid intake. Specify amount to be ingested in 24 hours, quantifying desired intake during the day, evening, and night shifts.

Offer fluid of patient's choice at bedside.

Instruct patient to inform nurse of thirst.

Review electrolytes, and report any abnormalities, especially Na^+, K^+, chloride, BUN, creatinine, hemoglobin, and hematocrit.

Confer with physician regarding need for parenteral electrolyte replacement therapy.

Report and document output over ___ cc.

Report and document output under ___ cc.

Evaluate presence of weakness during activity, and pace activity according to patient's tolerance.

Limit activity to reduce active bleeding. Specify limitation.

Other interventions specific to patient (specify).

Fluid Volume Deficit, High Risk

Related factors: Extremes of age, Extremes of weight, Excessive losses through normal routes, e.g., diarrhea, Loss of fluid through abnormal routes, e.g., indwelling tubes, Deviations affecting access to or intake or absorption of fluids, e.g., physical immobility, Factors influencing fluid needs, e.g., hypermetabolic state, Knowledge deficit related to fluid volume, Medications, e.g., diuretics, Others specific to patient (specify).

Definition: The state in which an individual is at risk of experiencing vascular, cellular, or intracellular dehydration (NANDA).

■ Suggested alternative diagnosis

Fluid Volume Deficit

■ Patient outcomes

Patient is oriented to person, place, and time.

Patient has moist mucous membranes.

Patient's vital signs are within normal limits for patient. Specify normal limits.

Patient's serum electrolytes, hemoglobin, and hematocrit are within normal range for patient. State normal range.

Patient's urine is less concentrated. Specify baseline specific gravity.

Patient reports no thirst.

Patient reports no weakness.

Other outcomes specific to patient (specify).

■ **Nursing interventions**

Assess and document skin turgor and mucous membranes q___ as parameters for adequate hydration.

Assess and document specific gravity and color or urine q___.

Assess and document color, amount, and frequency of emesis, diarrhea, and other drainage.

Assess and document vital signs q___.

Assess and document orientation to person, place, and time q___.

Assess and document dressing changes to evaluate fluid loss from wounds.

Assess and document skin temperature, dryness and color.

Assess and document intake and output.

Assess and document for active bleeding. Specify location.

Identify contributing factors that may aggravate dehydration, such as medications, fever, stress, medical orders.

Weigh patient q___. Baseline weight is ___.

Encourage oral fluid intake. Specify amount to be ingested in 24 hours, quantifying desired intake during the day, evening, and night shifts.

Offer fluid of patient's choice at bedside.

Instruct patient to inform nurse of thirst.

Review electrolytes, and report any abnormalities, especially Na^+, K^+, chloride, BUN, creatinine, hemoglobin, and hematocrit.

Limit activity to reduce active bleeding. Specify limitation.

Other interventions specific to patient (specify).

Fluid Volume Excess

Related factors: Increased fluid intake secondary to excess sodium, hyperglycemia, medications, compulsive water drinking, and so on; Insufficient protein secondary to decreased intake or increased losses; Decreased urine output secondary to renal dysfunction, heart failure, sodium retention, immobility, and so on, Others specific to patient (specify).

Definition: The state in which an individual experiences increased fluid retention and edema (NANDA).

■ **Defining characteristics**

Shortness of breath
Orthopnea
Rales
Oliguria
Uremia
Weight gain
Blood pressure change
Edema
Taut, shiny skin
Decreased urine output
Intake greater than output
Agitation, restlessness
Change in mental status
Change in respiratory pattern

Increased abdominal girth
Abnormal laboratory values (hematocrit, hemoglobin, sodium, chloride, protein)
Decrease in urine specific gravity
Neck vein distention
Abnormal breath sounds
Increase in central venous pressure, pulmonary artery pressure, pulmonary wedge pressure
Pleural friction rub
Presence of S3 heart sound
Effusion
Anasarca

■ **Suggested alternative diagnoses**

None

■ **Patient outcomes**

Patient's edema decreases toward normal limits for patient. Specify normal limits for patient.
Patient's target weight is achieved. Specify target weight.
Patient's skin integrity is maintained.
Patient verbalizes understanding of fluid and dietary restrictions.
Patient verbalizes understanding of prescribed medications.
Patient's vital signs are within normal limits for patient. Specify normal limits.
Other outcomes specific to patient (specify).

■ **Target date**

Specify estimated date of completion.

■ **Documentation interval**

Specify frequency.

■ Nursing interventions

Assess and document vital signs q ___.

Assess and document patient's weight q ___.

Assess and document intake and output q ___.

Assess, palpate, and document presence of edema (peripheral, sacral, periorbital). Specify location and degree of edema on scale from 1+ to 4+.

Assess and document abdominal girth q ___.

Assess edematous extremity or body part for impaired circulation and skin integrity, and document q ___.

Assess and document effects of medications on edema (such as steroids, diuretics, lithium).

Assess and document pulmonary and/or cardiovascular complications as indicated by increased respiratory distress, increased pulse rate, increased blood pressure, abnormal heart sounds, and/or abnormal lung sounds.

Monitor electrolytes, and report abnormalities to physician.

Elevate extremities to increase venous return.

Change position q ___.

Maintain patient's fluid restriction.

Instruct and encourage dietary restrictions.

Instruct patient on use, dosage, and side-effects of prescribed medication.

Instruct patient on causes and resolutions of edema.

Other interventions specific to patient (specify).

Gas Exchange, Impaired

Related factors: Decreased pulmonary blood supply secondary to pulmonary hypertension, pulmonary embolus, congestive heart failure, respiratory distress syndrome, anemia, Decreased functional lung tissue secondary to chronic lung disease, pneumonia, thoracotomy, atelectasis, respiratory distress syndrome, mass, diaphragmatic hernia, Ventilation-perfusion imbalance, Others specific to patient (specify).

Definition: The state in which the individual experiences a decreased passage of oxygen and/or carbon dioxide between the alveoli of the lungs and the vascular system (NANDA).

■ Defining characteristics

Inability to move secretions
Confusion
Restlessness
Somnolence
Irritability
Hypoxia
Hypercapnia

■ Suggested alternative diagnoses

Airway Clearance, Ineffective
Breathing Pattern, Ineffective
Dysfunctional Ventilatory Weaning Response (DVWR)

■ Patient outcomes

Arterial blood gases are within normal limits for patient.
Pulmonary function is within normal limits for patient.
Patient is able to describe plan for care at home.
Other outcomes specific to patient (specify).

■ Target date

Specify estimated date of completion.

■ Documentation interval

Specify frequency.

■ Nursing interventions

Correlate all assessment data (patient sensorium, breath sounds, respiratory pattern, ABGs, sputum, effect of medications). Document and report any changes.

Increase frequency of monitoring when patient appears somnolent.

Consult with physician regarding future need for ABG test and use of supportive equipment as indicated by a change in the patient's condition.

Explain proper use of supportive equipment (oxygen, suction, spirometer, IPPB).

Assess patient's lung sounds, respiratory rate, and production of sputum as indicators of effective use of supportive equipment.

Reduce potential for increased oxygen consumption by reducing fever, decreasing pain, lessening anxiety, and pacing activity.

Pace activities to minimize fatigue and shortness of breath.

Inform patient before beginning intended procedures to lower anxiety and increase sense of control.

Reassure patient during periods of respiratory distress and/or anxiety.

Instruct patient in breathing and relaxation techniques to improve breathing pattern.

Explain to patient and family the reasons for low-flow oxygen by nasal cannula or mask when oxygen is required.

Inform patient and family that smoking is prohibited in room.

A suggested plan of care for a patient on a ventilator may include:

Verifying correct placement of ET tube.

Maintaining patent airway by suctioning patient and keeping an ET tube or trach replacement at bedside.

Ensuring effective breathing pattern by assessing for synchronization and possible need for sedation.

Ensuring adequate oxygen delivery by reporting abnormal ABGs, having ambu bag attached to oxygen source at bedside, and hyperoxygenating prior to suctioning.

Monitoring for complications (pneumothorax, unilateral aeration).

Instruct patient and family in plan for care at home (medications, activity, supportive equipment, reportable signs and symptoms, community resources).

Other interventions specific to patient (specify).

Grieving, Anticipatory

Related factors: Potential loss of significant person, animal, or prized material possession, Potential loss of body parts or functions, Impending death of self, Potential loss of social role, Others specific to patient (specify).

Definition: A state in which an individual grieves before an actual loss (NANDA).

■ Defining characteristics

Normal grieving initiated on anticipation of a significant loss
Denial
Shock
Disbelief
Physiologic symptoms, e.g., exhaustion, sighing, choking sensation, tightness in throat, changes in eating habits
Anger
Guilt
Sense of unreality
Altered sleep pattern
Sorrow, weeping
Altered activity level
Altered libido
Altered communication patterns
Hope that loss can be prevented

■ Suggested alternative diagnosis

Grieving, Dysfunctional

■ Patient outcomes

Patient/family expresses thoughts and feelings regarding anticipated loss.
Patient/family participates in grief work.
Patient/family demonstrates ability to make mutual decisions regarding anticipated loss.
Patient/family uses appropriate resources.
Other outcomes specific to patient/family (specify).

■ Target date

Specify estimated date of completion.

■ Documentation interval

Specify frequency.

■ **Nursing interventions**

Assess past experience of patient/family with loss, existing support systems, current grief work.

Respect culture, religion, race, and values of patient/family as patient/family expresses grief.

Help patient/family to share mutual fears, plans, concerns, and hopes with each other.

Assist patient/family to verbalize fears/concerns of potential loss.

Discuss the phases of the grieving process with patient/family.

Discuss with patient/family the impact of anticipated loss on the family unit and its functioning.

Refer to appropriate resources. Consider support groups, legal assistance, financial assistance, social services, religious/spiritual assistance.

Other interventions specific to patient/family (specify).

Grieving, Dysfunctional

Related factors: Actual loss (specify), Anticipated loss (specify), Chronic illness, Perceived loss (specify; objects may include: people, possessions, a job, status, home, ideals, parts and processes of the body), Terminal illness, Others specific to patient (specify).

Definition: A state in which an individual reacts to an actual, anticipated, or perceived loss of a significant person, ideal, status, object, or body part with an absent, delayed, exaggerated, or prolonged response.

■ Defining characteristics

Expressing distress at loss
Denial of loss
Expressing guilt
Expressing unresolved issues
Anger
Sadness
Crying
Alteration in eating habits
Alteration in sleep patterns
Alteration in activity level

Developmental regression
Labile affect
Alteration in concentration and/or pursuits of tasks
Difficulty in expressing loss
Alteration in dream patterns
Alteration in libido
Idealization of lost object
Reliving past experiences
Interference with life functioning

■ Suggested alternative diagnoses

Adjustment, Impaired
Coping, Ineffective Individual
Grieving, Anticipatory
Thought Processes, Altered

■ Patient outcomes

Patient demonstrates independence in activities of daily living.
Patient verbalizes grief.
Patient shares grief with significant person.
Patient verbalizes meaning of loss.
Patient participates actively in decision-making process.
Patient uses available support systems.
Other outcomes specific to patient (specify).

■ Target date

Specify estimated date of completion.

■ Documentation interval

Specify frequency.

■ **Nursing interventions**

Assess and document the presence and source of patient's grief.

Avoid confrontation of denial, and at the same time do not reinforce denial.

Balance any misperceptions with reality.

Establish a trusting relationship with patient and family.

Encourage patient to express grief.

Discuss the phases of the grieving process with patient.

Evaluate verbal and nonverbal communication as they relate to grieving process.

Provide a safe, secure, and private environment to facilitate patient/family grieving process.

Recognize and reinforce the strength of each family member.

Acknowledge patient's and family's grief reactions while continuing necessary care activities. Allow for flexibility in schedule of activities.

Encourage independence in performance of self-care, assisting patient only as necessary.

Help patient/family to participate actively in decision-making process.

Demonstrate respect for patient's culture, religion, race, and values as patient expresses grief.

Discuss with patient/family the impact of the loss on the family unit and its functioning.

Seek support among peers and others to provide patient care as needed.

Provide patient/family with information about hospital and community resources, such as self-help groups.

Initiate a patient care conference to review patient/family needs related to their state of the grieving process and to establish a plan of care. Support provided by ___.

Establish a schedule for contact with patient. Interact with patient q ___. Document contact.

Other interventions specific to patient (specify).

Growth and Development, Altered

Related factors: Inadequate prenatal care, Congenital anomaly, Fetal distress during or after birth/delivery, Prematurity, Neonatal disease, Unhealthy maternal lifestyle during pregnancy, Maternal acute/chronic disease, Maternal age, Inadequate caretaking, Poverty, Changes in family system, Inadequate bonding, Lack of stimulation in environment, Abuse, Traumatic separation, Loss, Rapid growth, Serious illness/injury, Prescribed dependence/limitations, Indifference, Inconsistent responsiveness, Multiple caretaking, Separation from significant others, Environment and stimulation deficiencies, Effects of physical disability, Prescribed dependence, Others specific to patient (specify).

Definition: The state in which an individual demonstrates deviations in norms from his/her age group (NANDA).

■ **Defining characteristics**

Major

Delay or difficulty in performing skills (motor, social, or expressive) typical of age group
Altered physical growth
Inability to perform self-care or self-control activities appropriate for age

Minor

Flat affect
Listlessness
Decreased responses
Infant irritability

■ **Suggested alternative diagnoses**

Coping, Ineffective Individual
Rape-Trauma Syndrome: Silent Reaction
Role Performance, Altered

■ **Patient outcomes**

Patient achieves the highest level of wellness, development, and independence possible, given patient's illness/disability.
Other outcomes specific to patient (specify).

■ **Target date**

Specify estimated date of completion.

■ **Documentation interval**

Specify frequency.

■ Nursing interventions

Establish a therapeutic and trusting relationship with caretakers.

Conduct a thorough health assessment (e.g., child's history, temperament, culture, family environment, developmental screening) to determine functional level.

Create an environment where ADLs can be performed with maximum independence.

Assist patient in achieving next level of growth and development through appropriate mastery of tasks specific to his/her level.

Identify potential related physical problems (e.g., dehydration, falls, URI, skin breakdown), and initiate plans to prevent them.

Assess the caretakers' knowledge, resources, support system, coping skills, and level of commitment to develop a plan of care. (For possible care plans/interventions, refer to *Coping, Family: Potential for Growth; Coping, Ineffective Family: Compromised;* and *Coping, Ineffective Family: Disabling.*)

Act as case manager to assure comprehensive care by coordinating medical, school, rehabilitation, and social services.

Help the family develop a strategy to integrate the patient as an accepted member of the family and community.

Other interventions specific to patient (specify).

Health Maintenance, Altered

Related factors: Religious beliefs, Cultural beliefs, Lack of material resources, Lack of social supports, Motor impairment, Lack of ability to make deliberate and thoughtful judgments, Lack of or significant alteration in communication skills, Perceptual/cognitive impairment (complete/partial lack of gross and/or fine motor skills), Ineffective individual coping, Dysfunctional grieving, Unachieved developmental tasks, Ineffective family coping, Disabling spiritual distress, Others specific to patient (specify).

Definition: A state in which an individual is unable to identify, manage, and/or seek out help to maintain health (NANDA).

■ Defining characteristics

Limited use of health care agencies and personnel
Expressed desire to improve health behaviors
Limited use of preventive health measures
History of untreated, chronic symptoms of disease process
Unwillingness to improve health behaviors
Lack of finances, equipment, and/or social resources
Need to adhere to cultural/religious beliefs
Demonstrated lack of knowledge regarding basic health practices
Inability to take responsibility for meeting basic health practices
History of lack of health-seeking behavior

■ Suggested alternative diagnoses

Adjustment, Impaired
Denial, Ineffective
Noncompliance (specify)
Therapeutic Regimen Management, Ineffective Individual

■ Patient outcomes

Patient acknowledges adverse effects of health beliefs.
Patient acknowledges need for assistance after discharge.
Patient verbalizes willingness to follow nursing/medical regimen.
Patient verbalizes knowledge of preventive health measures.
Other outcomes specific to patient (specify).

■ Target date	■ Documentation interval
Specify estimated date of completion.	Specify frequency.

■ Nursing interventions

Identify deficits that interfere with health maintenance. Specify.

Identify beliefs that interfere with health maintenance. Specify.

Provide a nonjudgmental environment in which patient/family can share beliefs.

Initiate a multidisciplinary patient care conference to plan health maintenance program with patient and family. Plan is ___ (specify).

Encourage discussion of preventive health measures specific to patient needs, such as dietary changes, cessation of smoking, stress reduction, and implementation of exercise program.

Offer information on community resources specific to health maintenance needs of patient/family.

Consult with social services to plan for health maintenance needs on discharge.

Other interventions specific to patient (specify).

Health-Seeking Behaviors *(specify)*

Related factors: Specific to patient.

Definition: A state in which a patient in stable health is actively seeking ways to alter personal health habits and/or the environment in order to move toward optimal health (NANDA).

■ **Defining characteristics**

Major	*Minor*
Expressed or observed desire to seek a higher level of wellness	Stated or observed unfamiliarity with wellness community resources
	Expressed or observed desire for increased control of health practice
	Demonstrated or observed lack of knowledge of health-promoting behaviors
	Expressed concern about current environmental conditions on health status

■ **Suggested alternative diagnoses**

Breast-Feeding, Effective (Potential for Enhanced)
Coping, Family: Potential for Growth

■ **Patient outcomes**

Patient describes health-seeking/health-promoting behaviors.
Patient describes ways of attaining a higher level of health.
Patient utilizes wellness community resources.
Other outcomes specific to patient (specify).

■ **Target date**	■ **Documentation interval**
Specify estimated date of completion.	Specify frequency.

■ Nursing interventions

Assess patient/family level of knowledge about measures for preventing illness.

Assess patient/family level of knowledge of signs and symptoms of disease condition and controllable aspects of the disease.

Discuss with patient/family personal health habits, and determine which behaviors may be changed to achieve optimal health (diet, smoking cessation, stress reduction, exercise program).

Reinforce positive health-seeking behaviors.

Provide patient/family with information about available wellness community resources.

Consult with community services as a primary step toward health promotion for patient/family. Involve patient/family in consultation.

Assist patient/family in developing a plan for increased health-promoting activities.

Other interventions specific to patient (specify).

Home Maintenance Management, Impaired

Related factors: Physical impairment of family member other than patient, Home environment obstacles, Inadequate support system, Insufficient family organization or planning, Insufficient finances, Lack of familiarity with community resources, Developmental disability, Psychologic impairment (specify), Lack of knowledge (specify), Lack of role modeling, Lack of knowledge, Impaired cognitive or emotional functioning, Individual/family member disease or injury, Others specific to patient (specify).

Definition: A state in which an individual, family, or household member is unable to independently maintain a safe, growth-promoting immediate environment (NANDA).

■ **Defining characteristics**

Major

Family/household members describing financial crises

Family/household members expressing inability to maintain home in a comfortable fashion

Family/household members requesting assistance with home maintenance

Unwashed or unavailable cooking equipment, clothes, linen

Accumulation of dirt, food wastes, or hygienic wastes

Overtaxed (e.g., exhausted, anxious) family members

Repeated hygienic disorders, infestations, or infections

Minor

Presence of vermin or rodents

Disorderly surroundings

Offensive odors

Inappropriate household temperature

■ **Suggested alternative diagnoses**

None

■ **Patient outcomes**

Patient/family/household member describes plan to correct obstacles/hazards in home.

Patient/family household member verbalizes knowledge of available resources.

Patient/family/household member identifies options to overcome financial constraints.

Patient/family/household member follows specific plan for home maintenance.

Patient/family/household member verbalizes awareness of constraints on home situation due to illness of family member.

Other outcomes specific to patient/family/household member (specify).

■ **Target date**   ■ **Documentation interval**

Specify estimated date of completion.   Specify frequency.

■ **Nursing interventions**

Help patient/family/household member identify obstacles/hazards in home that may impede home maintenance.

Initiate discussion with patient/family about health status of all family members, as illness of other family members may affect home maintenance management.

Accept and support without judgment the realities of the home situation.

Contact discharge planning/social worker to establish realistic plan for home maintenance.

Involve patient/family/household member in all planning activities.

Help patient/family/household member identify strengths in family unit as well as support systems that will assist in home maintenance.

Provide patient/family/household member with written material regarding home maintenance.

Assess and document need for postdischarge follow-through with public health nurse.

Other interventions specific to patient/family/household member (specify).

Hopelessness

Related factors: Abandonment, Failing or deteriorating physical condition, Lack of social supports, Long-term stress, Lost spiritual belief, Prolonged activity restrictions creating isolation, Others specific to patient (specify).

Definition: A subjective state in which an individual sees no alternatives or personal choices available and cannot mobilize energy on own behalf (NANDA).

■ Defining characteristics

Major	*Minor*
Verbal cues such as "I can't," "I don't care," sighing	Alteration in sleep patterns
	Lack of initiative
Decreased verbalization	Decreased response to stimuli
Passivity	Decrease in appetite
Decreased affect	Lack of involvement in care/passive allowance of care
	Closing eyes
	Shrugging in response to speaker
	Avoidance of eye contact
	Decreased affect

■ Suggested alternative diagnoses

Coping, Ineffective Individual
Grieving, Dysfunctional
Powerlessness

■ Patient outcomes

Patient identifies personal strengths.
Patient initiates behaviors that may reduce feelings of hopelessness.
Other outcomes specific to patient (specify).

■ Target date

Specify estimated date of completion.

■ Documentation interval

Specify frequency.

■ Nursing interventions

Explore with patient factors that contribute to feelings of hopelessness.

Assess and document potential for suicide.

Obtain psychiatric consultation.

Institute suicide precautions as needed (for example, 24-hour attendant, room close to nurses' station, removal of potentially harmful objects from room).

Provide opportunities for patient to initiate interactions and activities.

Encourage active participation in group activities to provide opportunity for social supports and problem solving.

Spend time with patient to provide opportunity to explore alternative coping measures. Schedule q ___.

Involve family/significant person in treatment plan.

Provide positive reinforcement for behaviors that demonstrate initiative, such as eye contact, self-disclosure, reduction in amount of sleep time, self-care, increased appetite.

Provide information on community resources, such as community agencies, social agencies, self-improvement classes, stress-reduction classes, counseling. Specify.

Other interventions specific to patient (specify).

Hyperthermia

Related factors: Prolonged exposure to hot environment, Vigorous activity, Illness or trauma, Medication/anesthesia, Dehydration, Inability or decreased ability to perspire, Excessive clothing, Increased metabolic rate, Others specific to patient (specify).

Definition: A state in which an individual's body temperature is elevated above his/her normal range (NANDA).

■ Defining characteristics

Major	Minor
Increase in body temperature above normal range	Flushed skin
	Skin warm to touch
	Increased respiratory rate
	Tachycardia
	Seizures/convulsions
	Confusion
	Light-headedness
	Nausea

■ Suggested alternative diagnosis

Body Temperature, Altered: High Risk

■ Patient outcomes

Patient's temperature is restored to normal.
Patient/family demonstrates proper method of taking temperature.
Patient/family describes measures to prevent/minimize increase in body temperature.
Patient/family reports early signs and symptoms of hyperthermia.
Other outcomes specific to patient (specify).

■ Target date

Specify estimated date of completion.

■ Documentation interval

Specify frequency.

■ Nursing interventions

Monitor temperature q ___.

Remove excess clothing, and cover patient only with a sheet.

Use cooling measures: submerge in tepid bath; apply cool washcloths to axillae, groin, forehead, and nape of neck; use a circulating fan in patient's room; use a cooling blanket.

Encourage intake of oral fluids.

Administer antipyretics per doctor's order.

Instruct patient/family in measures for prevention and early recognition of hyperthermia.

Other interventions specific to patient (specify).

(See nursing interventions for *Body Temperature, Altered: High Risk* on page 17.)

Hypothermia

Related factors: Prolonged exposure to cool or cold environment, Trauma, Hypothyroidism, Damage to hypothalamus, Inability or decreased ability to shiver, Malnutrition, Inadequate clothing, Consumption of alcohol, Medications causing vasodilation, Decreased basal metabolic rate, Inactivity, Aging, Loss of subcutaneous fat, Immaturity of newborn's temperature regulatory system, Low birth weight, Others specific to patient (specify).

Definition: The state in which an individual's body temperature is reduced below normal range (NANDA).

■ **Defining characteristics[1]**

Mild	Moderate	Severe
Shivering	Shivering	Muscular rigidity
Apathy	Cardiac arrhythmias	Respirations 5/min
Confusion	Bradycardia	Decreased urine output
Disorientation	Cyanosis	Absent reflexes
Cold skin	Dilated pupils	Cardiac arrhythmias
Slurred speech		
Amnesia		
Pallor		
Piloerection (goose bumps)		
Tachycardia		
Hypertension		

■ **Suggested alternative diagnosis**

Body Temperature, Altered: High Risk

■ **Patient outcomes**

Patient's temperature is restored to normal.
Patient/family describes measures to prevent/minimize decrease in body temperature.
Patient/family verbalizes early signs and symptoms of hypothermia.
Other outcomes specific to patient (specify).

■ **Target date**   ■ **Documentation interval**

Specify estimated date of completion.   Specify frequency.

■ Nursing interventions

Take patient's temperature with a low-range thermometer.

Record baseline vital signs.

Place patient on cardiac monitor.

Provide warmth: dry clothing, heated blankets, mechanical heating devices, adjusted room temperature, hot water bottles, submersion in warm water, warm oral fluids as tolerated.

For severe hypothermia, assist physician with core-warming techniques (e.g., hemodialysis, peritoneal dialysis, colonic irrigation, intragastric balloon, inhalation rewarming).[2]

Instruct patient/family in measures for prevention and early recognition of hypothermia.

Other interventions specific to patient (specify).

(See nursing interventions for *Body Temperature, Altered: High Risk* on page 17.)

---

[1]Matz, R.: Hypothermia: Measures and countermeasures, *Hospital Practice* 1986, 21 (1A): 45–71.

[2]Reuler, J.: Hypothermia: Pathophysiology, clinical settings, and management, *Annals of Internal Medicine* 1978, 89: 519–527.

Infant Feeding Pattern, Ineffective

Related factors: Prematurity, Neurological impairment/delay, Oral hypersensitivity, Prolonged NPO, Anatomical abnormalities.

Definition: A state in which an infant demonstrates an impaired ability to suck or coordinate the suck-swallow response (NANDA).

■ Defining characteristics

Inability to initiate or sustain an effective suck
Inability to coordinate sucking, swallowing, breathing

■ Suggested alternative diagnoses

None

■ Patient outcomes

Infant maintains steady and acceptable weight gain.
Infant coordinates suck-swallow with respirations while maintaining heart rate and color.
Other outcomes specific to infant (specify).

■ Target date

Specify estimated date of completion.

■ Documentation interval

Specify frequency.

■ **Nursing interventions**

Assess infant's readiness for nipple feeding:
 Presence of rooting reflex (28–36 weeks).
 Gag reflex (32 weeks).
 Mature sucking reflex (32–34 weeks).
 Coordination of sucking, swallowing, and breathing (34 weeks).
 Neonatal Oral Motor Assessment Scale (NOMAS).
Refer to a physical or occupational therapist any infant who is not progressing with feeding or has structural or oral motor defects.
Determine most appropriate feeding method (nipple feeding, intermittent gavage, continuous feeding with NG tube, jejunal tube, or gastrostomy).
To increase success with nipple feeding:
 Provide consistent caregivers to better read infant's cues and facilitate infant learning; involve mother at earliest opportunity.
 Consider varying formula (thickness, taste, temperature).
 Choose most appropriate nipple (size, shape, firmness, size of hole).
 Feed the premature infant when fully alert and eager.
 Reduce light and noise levels.
 Establish regular respiration by calming the infant prior to feeding; during feeding remove nipple at first sign of respiratory or state changes.
 Remain relaxed and patient during feeding; allow brief rest periods; pace the infant to complete feeding in appropriate time (too quickly may compromise safety, too slowly may increase fatigue and calorie expenditure).
 Burp the infant frequently.
 Position the infant in a semi-upright position with head slightly forward and chin tilting down.
 Use facilitation techniques (prior to feeding, increase oral sensitivity by stroking the infant's lips, cheeks, and tongue; during feeding, place your fingers on each cheek and under the jaw midway between the chin and throat to provide inward and forward support of the cheeks and tongue).
 Avoid techniques that interrupt infant's learning by allowing passive flow of liquid without infant's active participation (twisting or jiggling bottle, moving nipple up and down, moving nipple in and out of infant's mouth, moving infant's jaw up and down).
 Overfill bottle above amount of scheduled feeding to make sucking easier and to minimize sucking of air.
At each feeding, assess infant's nipple feeding skills by evaluating if infant:
 Actively sucks liquid from bottle.
 Actively initiates swallow in coordination with suck.
 Loses minimal liquid from mouth.
 Completes feeding in acceptable time.
 Coordinates sucking, swallowing, and breathing.
At each feeding, assess respiratory function and behavioral state and monitor infant for problems such as regurgitation, abdominal distention, and increased residuals.

Daily assess whether the infant is ready to advance. Consider a feeding flow sheet to facilitate assessment; document infant's state, oxygen needs, preferred nipple, position, formula type/temperature, amount of feeding taken in first 10 minutes, total feeding, total feeding time, daily weight, and stool pattern.

Prior to discharge, assess mother's readiness to feed infant, teach feeding techniques and support her during feeding.

Arrange for home visit within 72 hours of discharge.

Establish support network to ensure that mother has help with day-to-day lactation/ breast-feeding problems as they occur.

Other interventions specific to infant (specify).

Infection: High Risk

Risk factors: Broken skin, Traumatized tissue, Decrease in ciliary action, Stasis of body fluids, Change in pH secretions, Altered peristalsis, Decreased hemoglobin, Leukopenia, Suppressed inflammatory response, Immunosuppression, Inadequate acquired immunity, Tissue destruction and increased environmental exposure, Chronic disease, Invasive procedures, Malnutrition, Pharmaceutical agents, Trauma, Rupture of amniotic membranes, Insufficient knowledge to avoid exposure to pathogens, Others specific to patient (specify).

Definition: The state in which an individual is at increased risk for being invaded by pathogenic organisms (NANDA).

■ Suggested alternative diagnoses

Home Maintenance Management, Impaired
Protection, Altered
Skin Integrity, Impaired: High Risk

■ Patient outcomes

Patient is free of signs and symptoms of infection.
Patient/family identifies signs and symptoms of infection.
Patient/family identifies factors that may increase the risk of infection.
Patient/family verbalizes willingness to alter life-style to decrease risk of infection.
Patient demonstrates adequate personal hygiene.
Other outcomes specific to patient (specify).

■ Target date	■ Documentation interval
Specify estimated date of completion.	Specify frequency.

■ Nursing interventions

Evaluate patient's risk for urinary, pulmonary, fungal, or viral infections.

Monitor patient for signs and symptoms of infection (consider temperature, pulse rate, drainage, appearance of wound, secretions, appearance of urine, skin temperature, skin lesions).

Monitor laboratory values (consider CBC, cultures, serum protein, and albumin).

Report suspicious findings to physician.

Protect patient from cross-contamination by not assigning same nurse to another patient with an infection, not rooming patient with an infected patient, limiting visitors as indicated, and providing protective isolation when indicated.

Instruct patient/family in signs and symptoms of infection, including elevated temperature, warm skin, wound warmth/redness/tenderness, unexpected drainage from wound site, generalized pain/discomfort, increased heart rate, localized swelling/redness/pain.

Explain to patient/family why illness and/or therapy increases the risk for infection.

Help patient/family identify factors in their environment, life-style, or health practices that increase risk of infection.

Refer patient/family to social services and/or community resources to assist patient/family in managing home, hygiene, nutrition.

Assist patient/family in beginning to make needed life-style changes, using whatever resources seem appropriate. Specify plan.

Instruct in and observe performance of personal hygiene practices to protect against infection.

Other interventions specific to patient (specify).

Injury: High Risk

Risk factors: *Internal: Biochemical, regulatory function:* Sensory dysfunction, Integrative dysfunction, Effector dysfunction, Tissue hypoxia, Malnutrition, Immune-autoimmune disorder, Abnormal blood profile, Leukocytosis/leukopenia, Sickle cell, Thalassemia, Decreased hemoglobin; *Physical:* Broken skin, Altered mobility; *Developmental age:* Physiologic, psychosocial factors; *Psychologic:* affective, orientation.

External: Biological: Immunization level of community, Microorganism; *Chemical:* Pollutants, Poisons, Drugs (pharmaceutical agents, alcohol, caffeine, nicotine, preservatives, cosmetics and dyes), Nutrients (vitamins, food types); *Physical:* Design, structure, and arrangement of community, building, or equipment; Mode of transport/transportation; People/provider; Noso-comial agents; Staffing patterns; Cognitive, affective, and psychomotor factors, Others specific to patient (specify).

Definition: A state in which the individual is at risk of injury as a result of environmental conditions interacting with the individual's adaptive and defensive resources (NANDA).

■ **Suggested alternative diagnoses**

Aspiration: High Risk
Home Maintenance Management, Impaired
Peripheral Neurovascular Dysfunction: High Risk
Poisoning: High Risk
Sensory/Perceptual Alterations: Visual, Auditory, Kinesthetic, Gustatory, Tactile, Olfactory (specify)
Skin Integrity, Impaired: High Risk
Suffocation: High Risk
Thought Processes, Altered
Tissue Perfusion, Altered: Peripheral
Trauma: High Risk
Violence, High Risk: Self-Directed or Directed at Others

■ **Patient outcomes**

Patient/family identifies risks that increase susceptibility to injury.
Patient/family identifies appropriate safety factors that protect individual/child from injury.
Patient verbalizes strategies that prevent injury.
Patient avoids physical injury.
Other outcomes specific to patient (specify).

■ **Target date**   ■ **Documentation interval**

Specify estimated date of completion.   Specify frequency.

■ **Nursing interventions**

Assess and document patient's motor and/or sensory deficit to determine safety needs of patient.

Assess and document degree of intoxication to determine safety needs of patient.

Assess and document changes in mental status to determine safety needs of patient.

Assess and document maturational age to determine safety needs of patient.

Assess high-risk areas that may lead to injury to patient/family.

Use pressure-reduction device, foot cradle, heel and elbow pads to prevent/inhibit further skin injury.

Reorient patient to reality and immediate environment when necessary.

Encourage patient to request assistance with activities.

Check patient for presence of constrictive clothing, cuts, burns, bruises.

Use heating devices with caution to prevent burns in patients with sensory deficit.

Do not support patient's hallucinations or otherwise contribute to disorientation.

Instruct patient/family in techniques to prevent injury at home (specify).

Instruct patient to use caution in use of heat therapy devices.

Explore strategies to prevent injury.

Provide educational materials related to strategies and countermeasures to prevent injury.

Provide information on environmental hazards and characteristics (e.g., stairs, windows, cupboard locks, swimming pools, streets, gates).

Refer to educational classes in the community.

Other interventions specific to patient (specify).

Knowledge Deficit *(specify)*

Related factors: Cognitive limitation, Information misinterpretation, Lack of motivation, Limited exposure to information (specify), Limited practice of skill (specify), Unreadiness to learn, Unfamiliarity with information resources, Lack of recall, Lack of interest in learning, Others specific to patient (specify).

Definition: A state in which the individual/family does not comprehend, learn, or demonstrate knowledge of health care measures necessary to maintain or improve health.

■ Defining characteristics

Verbalization of limited knowledge/understanding of health care measures
Inaccurate follow-through of instruction
Inaccurate performance on tests
Inappropriate or exaggerated behaviors (e.g., hysteria, hostility, agitation, or apathy)

■ Suggested alternative diagnoses

Adjustment, Impaired
Coping, Ineffective Individual
Denial, Ineffective
Health Maintenance, Altered
Noncompliance (specify)

■ Patient outcomes

Patient/family identifies need for additional information regarding prescribed treatment.
Patient/family verbalizes understanding of need for support services to ensure completion of learning.
Patient/family demonstrates ability to follow necessary health care measures.
Patient/family demonstrates ability to ___ (specify skill).
Other outcomes specific to patient/family (specify).

■ Target date   ■ Documentation interval

Specify estimated date of completion.   Specify frequency.

■ **Nursing interventions**

Assess and document patient's level of understanding of prescribed treatment.

Assess and document patient's readiness to learn treatment regimen.

Provide literature specific to patient's learning needs.

Develop a coordinated multidisciplinary teaching plan. Plan is ___ (specify).

Provide teaching at patient's level of understanding, repeating information as necessary. Be realistic.

Interact with patient in a nonjudgmental manner to facilitate learning.

Involve support person/family in teaching process.

Check for accurate feedback to ensure that patient understands prescribed treatment.

Document patient's progress in nurse's notes.

Plan with patient and physician adjustment in treatment to facilitate patient's ability to follow prescribed treatment.

Reinforce teaching as necessary, using multiple teaching approaches, return demonstrations, and verbal and written feedback.

Provide information on community resources that will help patient maintain treatment regimen.

Other interventions specific to patient (specify).

Mobility, Impaired Physical

Related factors: Pain/discomfort, Perceptual/cognitive impairment, Medically prescribed limitations, Musculoskeletal impairment, Neuromuscular impairment, Decreased strength and endurance secondary to ___, Depression/severe anxiety, Others specific to patient (specify).

Definition: A state in which the individual experiences a limitation of ability for independent physical movement (NANDA).

Level I: Independently uses equipment or device

Level II: Requires help from another person for assistance, supervision, or teaching

Level III: Requires help from another person and equipment/device

Level IV: Is dependent and does not participate in activity[1]

Specify level ___.

■ Defining characteristics

Reluctance to attempt movement
Impaired motor coordination, muscle strength
Limited range of motion
Inability to move purposefully within the physical environment
Imposed restrictions of movement, including mechanical and/or medical protocol

■ Suggested alternative diagnoses

Activity Intolerance
Unilateral Neglect

■ Patient outcomes

Patient verbalizes acceptance of limitations.
Patient demonstrates correct use of assistive devices with supervision.
Patient uses assistive devices correctly and independently.
Patient requests assistance with mobilization activities.
Patient performs mobilization activities with assistance.
Other outcomes specific to patient (specify).

■ Target date

Specify estimated date of completion.

■ Documentation interval

Specify frequency.

■ Nursing interventions

Assessment and documentation is an ongoing process to determine at which performance level patient's mobility is impaired.

Level I nursing interventions

Assistive device is ___ (specify).
Document patient's safe performance of activities with assistive devices.
Develop and document a plan for maintaining/increasing mobility. Plan is ___ (specify).
Provide positive reinforcement during activities.
Encourage patient/family to view limitations realistically.
Assess need for assistance from home health agency and need for durable medical equipment.
Other level I interventions specific to patient (specify).

Level II nursing interventions

Assist patient with mobility as necessary. Specify.
Supervise all mobilization attempts.
Document patient's safe performance of activities.
Develop and document a plan for maintaining/increasing mobility. (Use OT/PT as resource in planning patient care activities.) Plan is ___ (specify).
Assess patient's learning needs regarding ___ (specify).
Instruct patient in use of assistive device ___ (specify).
Instruct patient/family in ___ (specify).
Instruct and encourage patient in active/passive range-of-motion exercises to maintain or develop muscle strength and endurance.
Instruct the patient in safe transfer from bed to wheelchair or commode.
Instruct patient regarding weight-bearing status.
Instruct patient regarding correct body alignment.
Instruct and encourage patient to use a trapeze and/or weights to enhance and maintain strength of upper extremities.
Provide positive reinforcement during activities.
Assess need for assistance from home health agency and need for durable medical equipment.
Other level II interventions specific to patient (specify).

Level III and IV nursing interventions

Provide patient/family the opportunity to share feelings and concerns.
Encourage patient/family to view limitations realistically.
Provide positive reinforcement during activities.
Use OT/PT as resource in planning patient care activities.
Develop a plan to include the following:
    Active and passive range-of-motion exercises.
    Type of assistive device.
    Positioning of patient in bed/chair.
    Ways to transfer/turn patient.
    The number of personnel needed to mobilize patient.
    Necessary elimination equipment (bedpan/urinal/fracture pan).
    Schedule of activities.
    Maximization of patient's mobility, given necessary constraints.
Document patient's responses to plan.
Other level III and IV interventions specific to patient (specify).

Adapted from Jones, R., et al.: *Patient classification for long-term care: User's manual* (HEW Publication no. HRA-74-3107, November, 1974).

Noncompliance (specify)

Related factors: Denial of illness, Cultural beliefs, Spiritual beliefs, Dysfunctional relationship between client and provider, Negative consequence of treatment regimen, Negative perception of treatment regimen, Perceived benefits of continued illness, Others specific to patient (specify).

Definition: A person's informed decision not to adhere to a therapeutic recommendation (NANDA).

■ **Defining characteristics**

Major	Minor
Patient/family report of patient's noncompliance with treatment regimen	Failure to progress
	Failure to keep appointments
	Abnormal diagnostic test results
	Evidence of exacerbation of symptoms

■ **Suggested alternative diagnoses**

Adjustment, Impaired
Denial, Ineffective
Health Maintenance, Altered
Knowledge Deficit (specify)
Therapeutic Regimen Management, Ineffective Individual

■ **Patient outcomes**

Patient acknowledges consequences of continued noncompliant behavior.
Patient does not abuse health care providers physically or verbally.
Patient participates in the development of plan of care.
Patient follows agreed-on plan of care.
Other outcomes specific to patient (specify).

■ Target date	■ Documentation interval
Specify estimated date of completion.	Specify frequency.

■ Nursing interventions

Identify probable cause of patient's noncompliant behavior.

Encourage the patient to express feelings and concerns about hospitalization and relationship with health care providers.

Involve the patient in determining what behavior constitutes compliance.

Give positive reinforcement for compliance to encourage ongoing positive behaviors.

Develop a written contract with the patient, and evaluate compliant behaviors on a continuing basis. Contract is ___ (specify).

Inform patient that physical/verbal abuse is not acceptable and will not be tolerated.

Discuss with patient/family those factors that may have precipitated noncompliance with treatment regimen.

Initiate patient care conference to establish plan for consistent approach to patient. Plan is ___ (specify).

Communicate approach to all persons interacting with patient.

Evaluate patient's need for emotional support from hospital resources/social worker.

Provide emotional support to family members to help them maintain a positive relationship with patient.

Help patient/family to understand the need for following prescribed treatment and the consequences of noncompliance.

Consult with physician about possible alteration in medical regimen to encourage patient's compliance.

Other interventions specific to patient (specify).

Nutrition, Altered: Less Than Body Requirements

Related factors: Chemical dependence (specify), Difficulty in chewing, Difficulty in swallowing, Psychologic impairment (specify), Food intolerance, High metabolic needs, Lack of basic nutritional knowledge, Limited access to food, Loss of appetite, Nausea/vomiting, Inadequate sucking reflex in the infant, Parental neglect, Chronic illness, Economic factors, Others specific to patient (specify).

Definition: The state in which an individual experiences an intake of nutrients insufficient to meet metabolic needs (NANDA).

■ **Defining characteristics**

Abdominal pain
Difficulty in swallowing/chewing
Indigestion/stomach cramps
Aversion to eating
Alteration in taste sensation
Body weight 20% or more under ideal for height and frame
Refusal to eat
Weight loss with adequate food intake
Ulcerated oral mucosa
Diarrhea and/or steatorrhea
Hyperactive/hypoactive bowel sounds
Reported or evidence of lack of food
Satiety immediately after ingesting food
Perceived inability to ingest food
Inadequate food intake of less than recommended daily allowance
Pale conjunctival and mucous membranes
Poor muscle tone
Excessive loss of hair
Weakness of muscles required for swallowing or mastication
Capillary fragility
Lack of interest in food
Lack of information, misinformation
Misconceptions

■ **Suggested alternative diagnoses**

Breast-Feeding, Ineffective
Swallowing, Impaired
Therapeutic Regimen Management, Ineffective Individual

■ **Patient outcomes**

Patient maintains weight at ___ kg.
Patient describes components of nutritionally adequate diet.
Patient verbalizes willingness to follow diet.
Patient abstains from nonprescribed medication/substances.
Patient tolerates prescribed diet.
Patients gains ___ kg.
Other outcomes specific to patient (specify).

■ **Target date**	■ **Documentation interval**
Specify estimated date of completion.	Specify frequency.

■ **Nursing interventions**

Monitor and document food intake. Confer with physician regarding need for appetite stimulant, supplemental feedings, nutritional tube feedings, or TPN so that adequate caloric intake is maintained.
Assess and document bowel sounds and abdominal distention q ___.
Monitor laboratory values, especially transferrin, albumin, and electrolytes.
Weigh patient q ___.
Confer with dietitian to establish caloric requirements, especially for patients with high energy needs, such as those with burns, trauma, fever, and wounds, as well as postoperative patients.
Confer with dietitian to establish protein requirements for patients with inadequate protein intake or experiencing protein losses, such as patients with anorexia nervosa or glomerular disease/peritoneal dialysis.
Develop meal plan with patient to include schedule of meals, eating environment, patient likes/dislikes, food temperature.
Encourage family member to bring food of patient's preference from home.
Other interventions specific to patient (specify).

Difficulty in chewing/swallowing

Assess and document degree of swallowing difficulty.
Reassure patient, and provide calm atmosphere during meals.
Have suction catheters available at bedside, and suction during meals as needed.
Place patient in semi-Fowler's or high-Fowler's position to facilitate swallowing; have patient remain in this position for 30 minutes following meals to prevent aspiration.
Place food on unaffected side of mouth to facilitate swallowing.
When feeding patient, use syringe, if necessary, to facilitate swallowing.
Request occupational therapy consultation.

Nausea/vomiting

Identify factors precipitating nausea and vomiting.

Minimize factors that may precipitate nausea and vomiting. Specify.

Instruct patient in slow, deep breathing and voluntary swallowing to decrease nausea and/or vomiting.

Offer cool, wet washcloth to be placed on forehead or back of neck.

Ask patient to notify nurse of nausea.

Administer antiemetics on a set schedule to prevent nausea. Schedule is ___ (specify).

Document color, amount, and frequency of emesis.

Offer oral hygiene q ___.

Loss of appetite

Identify factors that may contribute to patient's loss of appetite (such as medications, emotional concerns).

Give positive feedback to patient who shows increased appetite.

Infant feeding

Assess mother's feeding techniques.

Instruct mother in feeding techniques that may increase baby's intake.

Use ___ nipples.

Feed baby on demand.

Provide privacy for mother and baby during feedings.

Feed baby q ___.

Monitor baby's intake. Confer with pediatrician regarding change in formula, change in schedule, supplemental feedings, and/or gavage feedings as appropriate.

Nutrition, Altered: More Than Body Requirements (Actual/High Risk)

Related factors/risk factors: Eating disorders (bulimia, binging), Increased appetite, Chemical dependence, Lack of physical exercise, Lack of basic nutritional knowledge, Ethnic/cultural norms, Decreased metabolic requirements, Excessive intake in relation to metabolic needs, Reported or observed obesity in one or both parents, Rapid transition across growth percentiles in infants or children, Reported use of solid food as major food source before 5 months of age, Observed use of food as reward or comfort measure, Reported or observed higher baseline weight at beginning of each pregnancy, Dysfunctional eating patterns, Pairing food with other activities, Concentrating food intake at end of day, Eating in response to external cues, e.g., time of day or social situation, Eating in response to internal cues other than hunger, e.g., anxiety, Others specific to patient (specify).

Definition (Actual): The state in which an individual is experiencing an intake of nutrients that exceeds metabolic needs (NANDA).

Definition (High Risk): The state in which an individual is at risk of experiencing an intake of nutrients that exceeds metabolic needs (NANDA).

■ Defining characteristics

Body weight 10–20% above ideal for height and frame
Triceps skinfold greater than 15 mm for men, 25 mm for women
Little or no exercise
Substituting sweets for addiction
Medications that stimulate appetite
Selecting foods that do not meet daily requirements
Dysfunctional eating patterns
    Pairing food with other activities
    Concentrating food intake at end of day
    Eating in response to external cues, such as time of day or social situation
    Eating in response to internal cues, such as anxiety, anger, depression, boredom, stress, loneliness
    Conforming to cultural norms

■ **Suggested alternative diagnosis**

Therapeutic Regimen Management, Ineffective Individual

■ **Patient outcomes**

Patient acknowledges weight problem.
Patient verbalizes desire to lose weight.
Patient participates in a structured weight-loss program.
Patient participates in a regular exercise program.
Patient approaches ideal weight.
Patient refrains from binge eating.
Other outcomes specific to patient (specify).

■ **Target date**	■ **Documentation interval**
Specify estimated date of completion.	Specify frequency.

■ **Nursing interventions**

Explore with patient/family factors that may be contributing to obesity.

Help patient to identify physical problems that may be related to obesity/eating disorder.

Monitor laboratory values that may be indicative of malnutrition (e.g., serum albumin, serum protein, transferrin).

Confer with dietitian to implement weight-loss/eating disorder program that includes dietary management and activity expenditure.

Develop a weight-loss plan to include:

    Two-week food and daily activity diary (amount, time, location, mood, social setting).

    Target weight loss.

    Self-monitoring.

    Education, e.g., causes of obesity, nutritional information, energy expenditure.

    Positive reinforcement.

    Behavior substitution.

    Exercise regimen.

    Anticipatory planning for social/business situations that include food.

    Group support.

    Strategies for control/avoidance of stimulus to eating.

Develop a plan for management of eating disorder to include:

    Frequency of meals and snacks.

    Diet of complex carbohydrates, protein.

    Avoidance of simple sugars, fast food, caffeine, soft drinks.

    Discussion of emotions that stimulate eating.

    Recognition of high-risk situations (types of foods, social situations, interpersonal stresses, unmet personal expectations, eating in secret/private).

    Behavior substitution.

    Group support.

Provide frequent positive reinforcement for weight loss, maintenance of dietary regimen, improved eating behaviors, exercise.

Instruct patient/family in food selection, preparation, and portions.

Provide information regarding available community resources, such as weight-loss groups, dietary counseling, exercise programs, self-help groups.

Other interventions specific to patient (specify).

Oral Mucous Membrane, Altered

Related factors: Inadequate oral hygiene, Chemotherapy, Lack of or decreased salivation, Medication, Infection, Malnutrition, Radiation to head and neck, Dehydration, NPO for more than 24 hours, Mouth breathing, Trauma (chemical, e.g., acidic foods, drugs, noxious agents, alcohol; mechanical, e.g., ill-fitting dentures, braces, tubes [nasogastric, endotracheal], surgery in oral cavity), Others specific to patient (specify).

Definition: The state in which an individual experiences disruptions in the tissue layers of the oral cavity (NANDA).

■ Defining characteristics

Discomfort with hot or cold foods
Oral pain/discomfort
Oral lesions or ulcers
Lack of or decreased salivation
Edema
Hyperemia
Oral plaque
Bad breath
Coated tongue
Dry, cracked lips
Dry mouth
Irritation, inflammation, or ulceration of oral mucosa
Dental caries
Leukoplakia
Vesicles
Hemorrhagic gingivitis
Stomatitis

■ Suggested alternative diagnoses

None

■ Patient outcomes

Patient is able to ingest foods and fluids with increasing comfort.
Patient performs essential oral hygiene according to prescribed instruction.
Patient has no increase in mucosal irritation, ulceration, or inflammation.
Other outcomes specific to patient (specify).

■ Target date

Specify estimated date of completion.

■ Documentation interval

Specify frequency.

■ Nursing interventions

Assess patient's oral mucosa for irritation, ulceration, and inflammation.

Identify substances that irritate oral mucosa, such as tobacco, alcohol, food, medication, extremes in food temperature, seasonings. Specify irritants.

Plan meals with patient and dietitian to ensure optimal nutrition and hydration.

Plan for oral care is ___ (specify). (Consider use of toothettes or soft child's toothbrush, bulb syringe, suction catheter, high-strength peroxide, and saline mouthwash.)

Assess and document patient's understanding of need for oral care and ability to perform oral care.

Instruct patient/family in routine for oral care.

Avoid use of commercial mouthwash, sugared candies, and gum.

Provide mouth care prior to meals and q ___ hours to ensure optimal oral hygiene and adequate nutrition.

Assist patient during meals as needed.

Monitor oral intake.

Clean dentures after each meal.

Confer with physician regarding an order for antifungal mouthwash or oral topical anesthetic as adjuncts to oral hygiene if fungal infection exits.

Other interventions specific to patient (specify).

Pain [Acute]

Related factors: Injury, Recent surgery, Noxious stimulus (specify), Others specific to patient (specify).

Definition: A state in which an individual reports discomfort or an uncomfortable sensation (adapted from NANDA). This discomfort is whatever the experiencing person says it is, existing whenever he/she says it does.[1]

■ **Defining characteristics**

Communication of pain descriptors, e.g., pain, discomfort, nausea, night sweats, muscle cramps, itching skin, numbness, tingling of extremities
Increased blood pressure
Increased/decreased pulse rate
Increased respiratory rate
Diaphoresis, pallor
Crying
Grimacing
Restlessness
Limited attention span
Withdrawal/focus on self
Guarding, protective behavior
Moaning
Pacing
Facial mask of pain
Alteration in muscle tone

■ **Suggested alternative diagnosis**

Pain, Chronic

■ **Patient outcomes**

Patient reports a decrease in pain.
Patient reports reasonable comfort.
Patient demonstrates individualized relaxation techniques that are effective for achieving comfort.
Patient's level of pain is maintained at ___ or less (scale of 0–10).
Other outcomes specific to patient (specify).

■ Target date	■ Documentation interval
Specify estimated date of completion.	Specify frequency.

■ **Nursing interventions**

Assessment

Use self-report as first choice to obtain assessment information.

If patient is preverbal or cognitively impaired, use family members for information.

In assessing patient's pain, use words that are consistent with patient's age and developmental level.[2]

Ask patient to rate pain/discomfort on a scale of 0–10 (0 = no pain/discomfort, 10 = worst pain). Document intensity of pain/discomfort.

Consider the impact of religion, culture, beliefs, and circumstances on patient's perception of pain/discomfort.

Assess nonverbal cues regarding level of pain/discomfort.

Complete initial pain assessment questionnaire (see p. 134).

Help patient identify comfort measures that have worked in the past, such as analgesics, distraction, relaxation, and application of heat/cold.

Explore feelings about fear of addiction. To reassure patient, ask, "If you didn't have this pain, would you still want to take this drug?"

Confer with physician on pain management, and assess need for change in pain medication order and use of nonpharmacologic interventions such as TENS and ice/heat application.

Document the pain-management plan.

Convey acceptance of patient's report of discomfort by a willingness to provide comfort measures.

Use pain flow sheet to monitor pain relief of analgesics and possible side effects (see p. 135). Adjust frequency of dosage as indicated.

Note that the elderly have increased sensitivity to analgesic effects of opiates, with higher peak effect and longer duration of pain relief.

Be alert to possible drug–drug and drug–disease interactions in the elderly, who often have multiple chronic, painful illnesses and take multiple medications.

Administer pain medication prior to activities/procedures.

Manage immediate post-operative pain with scheduled opiate (i.e., q4 hours for 36 hours) or patient-controlled analgesia (PCA).

Offer position change, back rubs, and relaxation techniques as supplements/alternative to medications for pain relief.

Change bed linen prn.

Encourage patient to maintain optimal activity level.

Provide care in an unhurried, supportive manner.

Involve patient in decisions regarding care activities.

Help patient focus on activities rather than on pain/discomfort by providing diversion through television, radio, tapes, and visitors.

Intervention

Explain reason for pain/comfort medication. Instruct patient to ask for pain/comfort medication before pain/discomfort becomes too severe.

Instruct patient to inform nurse if pain relief is not achieved.

Explain pain-management regimen to patient/family.

Inform patient of procedures that may increase pain, and offer suggestions for coping.

Instruct patient in use of sitz bath to increase comfort.

Include in discharge instruction: specific drug to be taken; frequency of drug administration; potential side effects; potential drug interaction; specific precautions to follow when taking the medication (e.g., physical activity limitations, dietary restrictions); name of person to notify about pain problem.

Other interventions specific to patient (specify).

---

[1]McCaffery, M.: *Nursing Management of the Patient with Pain,* 2nd ed. (Philadelphia: Lippincott, 1979).

[2]Acute Pain Management Guideline Panel. Acute pain management: Operative or medical procedure and trauma. *Clinical Practice Guideline.* AHCPR Pub. No. 92-0032. Rockville, MD: Agency for Health-Care Policy and Research, Public Health Service, U.S. Department of Health and Human Services, February, 1992.

Pain, Chronic

Related factors: Neurologic injury, Metastatic cancer, Altered body function (specify), Others specific to patient (specify).

Definition: A state in which an individual experiences pain that continues for more than 6 months in duration (NANDA). This pain is whatever the experiencing person says it is, existing whenever he/she says it does.[1]

■ **Defining characteristics**

Major	*Minor*
Verbal report or observed evidence of pain existing more than 6 months after expected time of healing/ discomfort	Frustration
	Depression
	Nausea
	Facial mask
	Guarded movements
	Fear of drug addiction
	Fear of drug tolerance
	Fear of reinjury
	Altered ability to continue previous activities
	Changes in sleep pattern
	Withdrawal, physical and social
	Weight changes

■ **Suggested alternative diagnosis**

Pain [Acute]

■ **Patient outcomes**

Patient reports reasonable comfort.
Patient reports increasing ability to cope with pain.
Patient verbalizes knowledge of alternative measures for pain relief.
Patient's level of pain is maintained at ___ or less (scale 0–10).
Other outcomes specific to patient (specify).

■ **Target date**	■ **Documentation interval**
Specify estimated date of completion.	Specify frequency.

■ **Nursing interventions**

Assessment

Use self-report as first choice to obtain assessment information. If patient is preverbal or cognitively impaired, use family members for information.

Ask patient to rate pain on a scale of 0–10 (0 = no pain and 10 = worst pain). Document patient's report of pain intensity.

Complete initial pain assessment questionnaire (see p. 134).

Be alert to verbal and nonverbal cues regarding level of pain experienced by the patient.

Assess and document effects of long-term medication use.

Intervention

Convey acceptance of patient's report of discomfort by a willingness to provide comfort measures.

Assist patient in identifying reasonable and acceptable level of pain.

Initiate a multidisciplinary patient care conference to develop a plan to manage discomfort. Plan should include identification and treatment of each symptom and its cause.

Use pain flow sheet to monitor pain relief and side effects (see p. 135).

Document patient's response to pain-relief measures.

Consult with physician for orders regarding alternative pain-relief measures, such as TENS, biofeedback, ice/heat application.

Offer patient pain-relief measures to supplement pain medication, such as biofeedback, relaxation techniques, back rub, and guided imagery.

Provide care in an unhurried, supportive manner, allowing for sufficient rest periods.

Incorporate patient's methods of pain relief in care.

Teaching

Convey to patient that total pain relief may not be achievable.

Instruct patient to inform nurse if desired pain relief is not achieved.

Instruct patient/family in use of alternative pain-relief measures.

Explain home pain-management regimen to patient/family.

Include in discharge instruction: specific drug to be taken; frequency of drug administration; potential side effects; potential drug interaction; specific precautions to follow when taking the medication (e.g., physical activity limitations, dietary restrictions); name of person to notify about pain problem.

Other interventions specific to patient (specify).

---

[1]McCaffery, M: *Nursing Management of the Patient with Pain,* 2nd ed. (Philadelphia: Lippincott, 1979).

El Camino Hospital

INITIAL PAIN ASSESSMENT

Dear Patient,

This questionnaire has been developed for you to describe your pain. Answer the questions as best you can - there are no right or wrong answers. A treatment plan will be written to help you achieve an acceptable level of comfort.

1. Please mark with an "X" on the drawing where you have pain.

2. On a scale of 0-10, if 0 was no pain and 10 the worst pain imaginable, rate your pain. Put your rating next to your "X" on the diagram.

3. Using the same pain scale, what level of pain would be acceptable to you at this time? (0 is no pain and 10 is the worst pain imaginable).

```
0   1   2   3   4   5   6   7   8   9   10
```

4. Describe your pain in your own words.

_____

_____

_____

5. Does your pain come and go?   Yes   No

6. Does your pain spread?   Yes   No
   Explain _____

_____

7. How long have you been having this pain? _____

8. What causes or increases your pain? _____

9. What do you do at home to make yourself more comfortable? _____

_____

10. When you experience pain, do any of the following occur:

What helps to relieve these symptoms?

____ change in appetite _____

____ nausea and vomiting _____

____ constipation _____

____ difficulty urinating _____

____ coughing _____

____ change in breathing _____

____ dizziness _____

____ confusion _____

____ insomnia _____

____ depression _____

____ anger _____

____ anxiety _____

____ fatigue _____

____ change in ability to work _____

____ change in sexual function _____

Thank you for completing this questionnaire.   *Pain Management Task Force, 3/86*

Form 2041 (Rev. 6/86)

EL CAMINO HOSPITAL

Patient Label

PAIN FLOW SHEET

Purpose: To evaluate the safety and effectiveness of interventions and to maintain pain rating below patient's acceptable level of pain: _____.

DATE	TIME	*PAIN RATING	**INTERVENTION	PULSE	RESP.	BLOOD PRESSURE	LEVEL OF CONSCIOUSNESS/ OBSERVATIONS***	PLAN	COMMENTS/SIGNATURE

Adapted from McCaffery, M. 1982. Unpublished.

*Pain rating scale is 0-10, with 0 being no pain and 10 being the worst pain imaginable.

**For medications, include name, dose and route.

Pain Management Task Force, March, 1986.

Form 2042 7/86

***

Levels of consciousness:
1. awake, alert
2. awake, disoriented
3. sleepy, drowsy, needs verbal stimulation to stay awake
4. lethargic, needs to be shaken or moved to be aroused
5. responds only to pain

Parental Role Conflict

Related factors: Separation from child due to chronic illness; Intimidation with invasive or restrictive modality (i.e., isolation, intubation), specialized care centers or policies (e.g., apnea monitoring, postural drainage, hyperalimentation); Interruptions in family life due to home care regimen (treatments, caregivers, lack of respite); Change in marital status, career, roles; Relocation; Financial crisis, Legal crisis, Others specific to patient (specify).

Definition: The state in which a parent(s) who normally functions effectively experiences role confusion and conflict in response to crisis (adapted from NANDA).

■ **Defining characteristics**

Major	*Minor*
Expressed concern/feelings of inadequacy to provide for child's physical and emotional needs during hospitalization or in the home	Reluctance to participate in usual caretaking activities, even with encouragement and support
Demonstration of disruption in caretaking routines	Verbalization, demonstration of feelings of guilt, anger, fear, anxiety, and/or frustrations about effect of child's illness on family process
Expressed concerns about changes in parental role, family functioning, family communication, family health	
Expressed concern about perceived/actual loss of control over decisions relating to child	

■ **Suggested alternative diagnoses**

Caregiver Role Strain (Actual/High Risk)
Family Processes, Altered
Parenting, Altered
Parenting, Altered: High Risk

■ **Parent outcomes**

Parent(s) verbalizes desired parenting role.
Parent(s) demonstrates ability to modify parenting role in response to crisis.
Parent(s) expresses a sense of adequacy in providing for child's needs.
Other outcomes specific to parent (specify).

■ Target date	■ Documentation interval
Specify estimated date of completion.	Specify frequency.

■ Nursing interventions

Explain rationale for treatments, and encourage questions to minimize misunderstandings and maximize participation.

Ask parents to describe how they want to be involved in the care of their hospitalized child.

Give positive reinforcement for constructive parental actions.

Develop a plan of care involving parents. Consistently implement plan.

Confront parents with their ineffective parenting behaviors (during this crisis), and discuss alternatives.

Discuss with parent(s) a strategy for meeting personal/family's current needs.

Refer to community resources, support groups, social services.

Other interventions specific to parent (specify).

Parenting, Altered

Related factors: Absent or ineffective role model; Interruption in bonding process; Lack of knowledge/skill (specify); Lack of or inappropriate response of child to parent; Lack of support for nurturing figure(s); Psychologic impairment (specify); Unrealistic expectations of self, infant, partner; Dysfunctional relationship between parents/nurturing figures; Unmet maturational needs of parent; Physical/emotional abuse of parent; Significant stress (specify); Substance abuse (specify); Lack of cognitive functioning; Others specific to parent (specify).

Definition: The state in which a nurturing figure experiences an inability to create an environment which promotes the optimum growth and development of another human being (NANDA).

■ Defining characteristics

Major	*Minor*
Reported history of child abuse or abandonment by primary caretaker	Expressed disappointment with child
	Verbalization of resentment toward child
Inattentiveness to child's needs	Child out of control
Reluctant/inappropriate caretaking behaviors (toilet training, sleep/rest, feeding, discipline)	Avoidance of contact with child
	Noncompliance with health appointments for child
Evidence of physical and/or psychologic trauma to child	Frequent accidents/illnesses
	Growth and development lag
	Compulsive seeking of role approval from others
	Child receiving care from multiple caretakers without consideration of needs of the infant/child

■ Suggested alternative diagnoses

Caregiver Role Strain (Actual/High Risk)
Coping, Ineffective Family: Disabling
Family processes, Altered
Parenting, Altered: High Risk
Role Performance, Altered

■ Parent outcomes

Parent(s) reports increasing confidence in care of child.
Parent(s) reports increasing confidence in parenting role.
Parent(s) demonstrates nurturing behaviors toward child, including constructive discipline.
Parent(s) identifies effective ways to express anger/frustration that are not harmful to child.
Parent(s) identifies community resources that assist with home care.
Parent(s) actively participates in counseling.
Parent(s) participates in parenting classes.
Other outcomes specific to parent (specify).

■ Target date   ■ Documentation interval

Specify estimated date of completion.   Specify frequency.

■ Nursing interventions

Acknowledge and reinforce parenting strengths and skills.
Help parent identify deficits/alterations in parenting skills.
Encourage expression of feelings (guilt, anger, ambivalence) regarding parenting role.
Initiate a plan to assist parent in developing/adapting parenting skills. Consider:
    Frequent opportunities for parent/child interaction.
    Role modeling of parenting skills of nurse.
    Identifying realistic expectations of parenting role.
Explore available resources with parent.
Offer to make initial telephone call to appropriate community resources.
Report actual or suspected child abuse to appropriate authority.
Request social service consultation to help the family identify sources of community support.
Develop a plan for meeting needs of parent. Plan may include counseling, support groups, and hot lines.
Other interventions specific to parent (specify).

Parenting, Altered: High Risk

Risk factors: Adult children of alcoholics, Unmet maturational needs of parent, Absent or ineffective role model, History of child abuse or abandonment of parent, Absence of or ineffective support system, Lack of knowledge regarding effective parenting, Poverty/homelessness, Perceived threat to parent's physical or emotional survival, Mental or physical illness/disability, Presence of significant stress, Lack of or inappropriate response of child to parent, Others specific to patient (specify).

Definition: Possibility of changes in ability of nurturing figure(s) to create an environment which promotes the optimum growth and development of another human being (NANDA).

■ Suggested alternative diagnosis

Caregiver Role Strain: High Risk

■ Parent outcomes

Parent(s) identifies own risk factors that may lead to ineffective parenting.
Parent(s) identifies high-risk situations that may lead to ineffective parenting.
Parent(s) uses identified resources to maintain/learn/improve parenting skills.
Parent(s) maintains satisfactory parenting role.
Other outcomes specific to parent (specify).

■ Target date	■ Documentation interval
Specify estimated date of completion.	Specify frequency.

■ Nursing interventions

Help parent(s) identify high-risk situations/factors that may hinder effective parenting.
Help parent(s) to develop strategies to maintain/learn/improve parenting skills.
Acknowledge and reinforce parenting strengths and skills.
Refer to community support/educational programs to assist with development of parenting skills and provide anticipatory guidance.
Provide reading material as appropriate.
Other interventions specific to parent (specify).

Peripheral Neurovascular Dysfunction: High Risk

Risk factors: Fractures, Mechanical compression, e.g., tourniquet, cast, brace, dressing or restraint, Orthopedic surgery, Trauma, Immobilization, Burns, Vascular obstruction.

Definition: A state in which an individual is at risk of experiencing a disruption in circulation, sensation, or motion of an extremity (NANDA).

■ **Suggested alternative diagnoses**

None

■ **Patient outcomes**

Patient/family verbalizes signs and symptoms of peripheral neurovascular dysfunction.
Patient/family describes measures to prevent development of neurovascular dysfunction.
Patient is free of injury from compression devices or restraints.
Patient demonstrates optimal healing and adaptation to cast, traction, or dressing.
Other outcomes specific to patient (specify).

■ Nursing interventions

Perform the following neurovascular assessments every hour for the first 24 hours
   following casting, injury, traction, or restraints. Then, if stable, q4 hours.
   Assess and document circulation (color, temperature, capillary refill, edema,
      and distal pulses) to involved extremity.
   Conduct systematic evaluation of the sensory function of the involved periph-
      eral nerve (interview patient for subjective symptoms, pinprick, parathesias).
   Assess motor function, movement, and strength of the involved peripheral
      nerve.
   Assess for and report increasing and progressive pain that is present on passive
      movement and not relieved by narcotics, which may be first sign of com-
      partment syndrome.
Avoid tight dressings and appliances to prevent ischemia.
Elevate involved extremity to increase venous return and minimize edema.
Listen to patients expressed complaints of pain, burning, and changes in sensation.
   Recognize that restlessness, fussiness, and crying may be nonverbal cues of physical
   distress in infants, children, or adults with impaired verbal communication.
Institute immediate treatment if compartment syndrome is suspected: keep involved
   extremity at heart level, notify physician, and anticipate removal of anterior cast,
   occlusive bandages, and surgical intervention.
Teach patient/family routine cast care and measures to prevent complications.
Teach patient/family signs and symptoms of peripheral nerve injury and importance
   of immediate medical attention (pain not relieved by medication, paresthesia of
   involved body part).
Emphasize importance of keeping follow-up appointments with physician.
Other interventions specific to patient (specify).

Personal Identity Disturbance

Related factors: Situational crisis (specify), Psychologic impairment (specify), Chronic illness, Chronic pain, Congenital defects, Others specific to patient (specify).

Definition: Alteration in one's ability to distinguish between the self (ego) and nonself (Adapted from NANDA).

■ **Defining characteristics**

Change in social involvement
Extension of body boundary to incorporate environmental objects
Grandiose behavior

■ **Suggested alternative diagnosis**

Thought Processes, Altered

■ **Patient outcomes**

Patient identifies personal strengths.
Patient acknowledges impact of situation on existing personal relationships/life-style/ role performance.
Patient maintains close personal relationships.
Patient verbalizes willingness to consider life-style change.
Patient expresses willingness to use suggested resources on discharge.
Other outcomes specific to patient (specify).

■ Target date	■ Documentation interval
Specify estimated date of completion.	Specify frequency.

■ **Nursing interventions**

Encourage patient to verbalize consequences of physical and emotional changes that have influenced self-concept.

Encourage patient to verbalize concerns about close personal relationships.

Actively listen to patient/family, and acknowledge reality of concerns about treatments, progress, and prognosis.

Request psychiatric consultation.

Encourage patient/family to air feelings and to grieve.

Provide care in a nonjudgmental manner, maintaining the patient's privacy and dignity.

Assist patient to identify personal strengths.

Help patient identify alternative behaviors that are congruent with a change in personal relationships, life-style, and/or role performance.

Develop a plan of care with patient/family that identifies coping mechanisms and personal strengths and acknowledges limitations. Specify plan.

Assess need for assistance from social services department for planning care with patient/family.

Offer to make initial phone call to appropriate community resources for patient/family.

Other interventions specific to patient (specify).

Poisoning: High Risk

Risk factors: *Internal (individual):* Reduced vision, Verbalization of occupational setting without adequate safeguards, Lack of safety or drug education, Lack of proper precautions, Cognitive or emotional difficulties; Insufficient finances.

External (environmental): Large supplies of drugs in house; Medicines stored in unlocked cabinets accessible to children or confused persons; Dangerous products placed or stored within the reach of children or confused persons; Availability of illicit drugs potentially contaminated by poisonous additives; Flaking, peeling paint or plaster in presence of young children; Chemical contamination of food and water; Unprotected contact with heavy metals or chemicals; Paint, lacquer, etc. in poorly ventilated areas or without effective protection; Presence of poisonous vegetation; Presence of atmospheric pollutants, Others specific to patient (specify).

Definition: Accentuated risk of accidental exposure to or ingestion of drugs or dangerous products in doses sufficient to cause poisoning (NANDA).

■ **Suggested alternative diagnosis**

Home Maintenance Management, Impaired

■ **Patient outcomes**

Patient/family identifies risks that increase possibility of poisoning.
Patient/family identifies and implements appropriate safety measures that protect individual/child from poisoning.
Patient/family develops strategies to prevent poisoning.
Patient/family implements use of countermeasures to protect self and others from injury.
Other outcomes specific to patient (specify).

■ **Target date**   ■ **Documentation interval**

Specify estimated date of completion.   Specify frequency.

■ Nursing interventions

Assess high-risk areas that may lead to injury to patient/family.

Explore strategies to prevent injury.

Provide educational materials related to strategies and countermeasures.

Provide information on environmental hazards and characteristics (e.g., stairs, windows, cupboard locks, swimming pools, streets, gates).

Provide information on Poison Control Center and exposure to medications and household products.

Refer to educational classes in the community (CPR, first aid, swimming classes).

Other interventions specific to patient (specify).

Post-Trauma Response

Related factors: Catastrophic illness, Accidents, Assault, Disaster, Participation in combat, Epidemic, Kidnapping, Rape, Terrorism, Torture, Others specific to patient (specify).

Definition: The state of an individual experiencing a sustained painful response to unexpected extraordinary life events (NANDA).

■ Defining characteristics

Major	*Minor*
Guilt about behavior required for survival	Emotional numbness
	Amnesia about traumatic event
Reliving the event; flashback	Reported difficulty with interpersonal relationships
Intrusive thoughts	
Repetitive nightmares or dreams	Sleep pattern disturbance
Survival guilt	Reported phobia regarding trauma
Excessive verbalization of traumatic event	Reported pronounced changes in sexual behavior
	Suicide attempt(s)
	Substance abuse
	Irritability
	Poor impulse control
	Withdrawal from activities and commitments

■ Suggested alternative diagnoses

Rape-Trauma Syndrome: Compound Reaction
Rape-Trauma Syndrome: Silent Reaction

■ Patient outcomes

Patient verbalizes feelings related to traumatic event.
Patient/family identifies community resources for postdischarge care.
Patient acknowledges value of counseling.
Other outcomes specific to patient (specify).

■ Target date

Specify estimated date of completion.

■ Documentation interval

Specify frequency.

■ Nursing interventions

Encourage patient to verbalize his/her account of the traumatic event.

Assess patient's potential for suicide.

Initiate suicide precautions.

Follow hospital/agency policy regarding legal responsibility for reporting to authorities.

Initiate a multidisciplinary patient care conference to develop a plan of care. Specify.

Involve family/significant person in treatment plan.

Encourage verbalization of concerns by using caregivers who have an established rapport with patient and are knowledgeable about, and comfortable with, exploration of patient concerns.

Enhance patient's feeling of safety:

Promote a caring and therapeutic relationship between patient and nurse.

Monitor/hold phone calls at patient's request.

Monitor/limit visitation.

Plan room assignment, considering private vs. semiprivate and choice of roommate.

Provide opportunities for patient to initiate interactions and activities.

Encourage active participation in group activities to provide opportunity for social supports and problem solving.

Support the patient needing an invasive medical procedure (which may precipitate flashbacks):

Explain necessity of procedure.

Stay with patient during procedure.

Encourage patient to discuss feelings after procedure.

Premedicate if needed to minimize distress/discomfort.

Provide information/referral on community resources (rape counselors, clergy, crisis centers, support groups, mental health professionals, social services, Victims' Assistance, Survivors of Trauma).

Other interventions specific to patient (specify).

Powerlessness

Related factors: Health care environment, Treatment regimen, Chronic illness, Terminal illness, Complications threatening pregnancy, Interpersonal interaction, Illness-related regimen, Life-style of helplessness, Others specific to patient (specify).

Definition: Perception that one's own action will not significantly affect an outcome; a perceived lack of control over a current situation or immediate happening (NANDA).

■ Defining characteristics

Severe

Verbal expressions of having no control or influence over situation
Verbal expressions of having no control or influence over outcome
Verbal expressions of having no control over self care
Depression over physical deterioration that occurs despite patient compliance with regimens
Apathy

Moderate

Nonparticipation in care or decision making when opportunities are provided
Expressions of dissatisfaction and frustration over inability to perform previous tasks and/or activities
Does not monitor progress
Expression of doubt regarding role performance
Reluctant to express true feelings
Fear of alienation from caregivers
Passivity
Inability to seek information regarding care
Dependence on others that may result in irritability, resentment, anger, and guilt
Does not defend self-care practices when challenged

Low

Expressions of uncertainty about fluctuating energy levels
Passivity

■ Suggested alternative diagnoses

Grieving, Dysfunctional
Hopelessness
Self-Esteem, Low: Chronic

■ **Patient outcomes**

Patient verbalizes feelings of powerlessness.
Patient identifies actions within his/her control.
Patient participates in decision making regarding plan of care.
Other outcomes specific to patient (specify).

■ Target date	■ Documentation interval
Specify estimated date of completion.	Specify frequency.

■ **Nursing interventions**

Use nurse/patient relationship to assist patient in expressing feelings about his/her situation.
Help patient to identify factors that may contribute to powerlessness.
Allow patient as much control over his/her situation as possible.
Involve patient in decision making about care routine.
Discuss with patient realistic options in care, providing explanations for these options.
Initiate a multidisciplinary patient care conference to discuss and develop patient care routine. Plan is ___ (specify).
Explain to patient the rationale for any change in the plan of care.
Provide flexibility in care regimen as needed by patient.
Other interventions specific to patient (specify).

Protection, Altered

Related factors: Extremes of age, Inadequate nutrition, Alcohol abuse, Abnormal blood profiles (e.g., leukopenia, thrombocytopenia, anemia, coagulation), Drug therapies (e.g., antineoplastic, corticosteroid, immune, anticoagulant, thrombolytic), Treatments (e.g., surgery, radiation), Diseases (e.g., cancer, immune disorders), Others specific to patient (specify).

Definition: The state in which an individual experiences a decrease in the ability to guard the self from internal or external threat such as illness or injury (NANDA).

■ **Defining characteristics**

Major	*Minor*
Deficient immunity	Chilling
Impaired healing	Perspiring
Altered clotting	Dyspnea
Maladaptive stress response	Cough
Neurosensory alteration	Itching
	Restlessness
	Insomnia
	Fatigue
	Anorexia
	Weakness
	Immobility
	Disorientation
	Pressure sores

■ **Suggested alternative diagnoses**

Infection: High Risk
Injury: High Risk
Peripheral Neurovascular Dysfunction: High Risk
Sensory/Perceptual Alterations: Visual, Auditory, Kinesthetic, Gustatory, Tactile, Olfactory (specify)
Skin Integrity, Impaired: High Risk

■ **Patient outcomes**

Patient/family verbalizes willingness to change behavior to decrease risk of injury/infection/bleeding.
Patient/family demonstrates behaviors that decrease risk of injury/infection/bleeding.
Patient is free of signs and symptoms of injury/infection/bleeding.
Patient/family identifies early signs and symptoms of injury/infection/bleeding.
Patient/family reports early signs and symptoms of injury/infection/bleeding.
Patient reports an increase in his/her ability to manage stress.
Other outcomes specific to patient (specify).

■ **Target date**   ■ **Documentation interval**

Specify estimated date of completion.   Specify frequency.

■ **Nursing interventions**

Prevention of infection
See nursing interventions for *Infection: High Risk* on page 107.

Prevention of injury
See nursing interventions for *Injury: High Risk* on page 109.

Prevention of bleeding
Evaluate extent of patient's bleeding risk.
Instruct patient to avoid trauma (e.g., from contact sports, sharp objects, stiff toothbrush).
Advise patient to wear medical identification bracelet and to alert dentist, physician.
Teach patient signs and symptoms of bleeding and when to report.
Teach patient first aid for bleeding.

Restoration and growth
Assist patient in achieving optimum sleep, rest, nutrition, activity, and stress management.
Discuss relaxation techniques with patient/family, and make appropriate referrals.
Consult dietitian for suggestions to improve nutrition.
Assist patient/family in identifying and planning an appropriate exercise program.
Provide information on community resources/support groups.
Explore with patient ways to enhance sleep/rest.
Confer with social services to identify appropriate referral for counseling.
Other interventions specific to patient (specify).

Rape-Trauma Syndrome

Related factor: Patient's biopsychosocial response to event.

Definition: The stress response pattern that occurs as a result of forcible or attempted forcible sexual penetration against the victim's will and consent. It includes an acute phase of disorganization of the victim's life-style and a long-term process of reorganization of life-style (adapted from NANDA).

- **Defining characteristics**

Acute phase (several weeks)

Emotional reactions
  Anger
  Embarrassment
  Fear of physical violence and death
  Self-blame
  Fear of pregnancy, sexually trans-
    mitted diseases
  Humiliation
  Revenge
  Suicidal/homicidal behavior
  Psychotic states
  Confusion
  Memory disturbance
  Inability to make decisions
Multiple physical symptoms
  GI irritability (e.g., stomach pains,
    appetite disturbance, nausea)
  GU disturbance (e.g., vaginal
    discharge, itching, burning on
    urination, generalized pain)
  Muscle tension (e.g., tension
    headaches and fatigue)
  Sleep pattern disturbance
    (e.g., hyperalertness, edginess,
    nervousness)
  Physical trauma (e.g., general
    soreness, bruises, lesions,
    trauma to mouth and rectum)

Reorganization phase

Life-style changes
  Changing residences
  Taking trips
  Seeking out family, friends for
    support
  Initiating period of celibacy
Emotional reactions
  Suicidal/homicidal behavior
  Psychotic states
  Promiscuity
  Use of alcohol/drugs
  Body image disturbance
Recurrent dreams and nightmares
  Reliving rape and victimization
  Symbolic dreams related to the rape
  Mastery dreams (indicate
    recovering)
Fears and phobias
  Fear of environment (location of
    rape/attempted rape)
  Fear of being alone
  Fear of crowds
  Sexual fears
  Fear of initiating/continuing rela-
    tionships that may lead to
    intimacy

- **Suggested alternative diagnoses**

Rape-Trauma Syndrome: Compound Reaction
Rape-Trauma Syndrome: Silent Reaction

■ **Patient outcomes**

Patient's symptoms of stress response are decreased.
Patient describes a plan that includes safety measures to reduce future risk.
Patient returns to previous level of biopsychosocial functioning.
Other outcomes specific to patient (specify).

■ **Target date**	■ **Documentation interval**
Specify estimated date of completion.	Specify frequency.

■ **Nursing interventions**

Approach patient in a nonjudgmental and supportive manner.
Allow adequate time for patient to respond to even simple questions.
Encourage patient to verbalize feelings.
Initiate rape protocol specific to health care facility re preservation of evidence, physical assessment, specimen collection, reporting to legal authorities, medical follow-up.
Treat physical injuries.
Assess need for hospitalization for physical or psychologic trauma.
Support and educate significant others. Encourage expression of feelings, and discuss therapeutic response to victim and changed behaviors.
Counsel immediate family, spouse, or partner to maintain close relationship with victim, with attention to dispelling feelings of blame (self or projected).
Assist patient/family to establish support network.
Identify with patient/family predictable behaviors in response to rape-trauma event.
Refer patient/family to rape crisis counseling.
Other interventions specific to patient (specify).

Rape-Trauma Syndrome: Compound Reaction

Related factors: Patient's biopsychosocial response to event.

Definition: The stress response pattern that occurs as a result of forcible or attempted forcible sexual penetration against the victim's will and consent. It includes an acute phase of disorganization of the victim's life-style and a long-term process of reorganization of life-style. In the compound reaction, previous psychiatric and/or medical conditions are reactivated (adapted from NANDA).

■ **Defining characteristics**

Acute phase (several weeks)

Emotional reactions
  Anger
  Embarrassment
  Fear of physical violence and death
  Self-blame
  Fear of pregnancy, sexually transmitted diseases
  Humiliation
  Revenge
  Suicidal/homicidal behavior
  Psychotic states
  Confusion
  Memory disturbance
  Inability to make decisions
Multiple physical symptoms
  GI irritability (e.g., stomach pains, appetite disturbance, nausea)
  GU disturbance (e.g., vaginal discharge, itching, burning on urination, generalized pain)
  Muscle tension (e.g., tension headaches and fatigue)
  Sleep pattern disturbance (e.g., hyperalertness, edginess, nervousness)
  Physical trauma (e.g., general soreness, bruises, lesions, trauma to mouth and rectum)
Signs of previous psychiatric conditions (acute psychosis, mania, major depression, suicidal behaviors, paranoia, delusions)
Signs of previous medical conditions
Alcohol and/or drug abuse

Reorganization phase

Life-style changes
  Changing residence
  Taking trips
  Seeking out family, friends for support
  Initiating period of celibacy
Emotional reactions
  Suicidal homicidal behavior
  Psychotic states
  Promiscuity
  Use of alcohol/drugs
  Body image disturbance
Recurrent dreams and nightmares
  Reliving rape and victimization
  Symbolic dreams related to the rape
  Mastery dreams (indicate recovering)
Fears and phobias
  Fear of environment (location of rape/attempted rape)
  Fear of being alone
  Fear of crowds
  Sexual fears
  Fear of initiating/continuing relationships that may lead to intimacy

■ **Suggested alternative diagnoses**

None

■ **Patient outcomes**

Patient safety is maintained during reactivation of psychiatric and/or medical conditions.

Patient discontinues use of alcohol/drugs.

Patient identifies the existence of a relationship between his/her own psychiatric and/or medical conditions and the rape episode.

Patient actively participates in rape counseling.

Patient returns to previous level of biopsychosocial functioning.

Other outcomes specific to patient (specify).

■ **Target date**	■ **Documentation interval**
Specify estimated date of completion.	Specify frequency.

■ **Nursing interventions**

Perform physical assessment based on patient's complaints to determine presenting medical conditions.

Perform psychosocial assessment that focuses on rape.

Assess and document patient's orientation to person, place, time, and situation.

Assess for suicidal ideation, and provide necessary safety precautions.

Correlate physical and psychosocial assessment data to determine patient's status.

Establish a plan of care to stabilize medical/psychologic condition to proceed with rape-trauma counseling.

Approach patient in a nonjudgmental and supportive manner.

Allow adequate time for patient to respond to even simple questions.

Encourage patient to verbalize feelings.

Support and educate significant others. Encourage expression of feelings, and discuss therapeutic response to victim and changed behaviors.

Counsel immediate family, spouse, or partner to maintain close relationship with victim, with attention to dispelling feelings of blame (self or projected).

Assist patient/family to establish support network.

Identify with patient/family predictable behaviors in response to rape-trauma event.

Refer patient/family to rape crisis counseling.

Other interventions specific to patient (specify).

Rape-Trauma Syndrome: Silent Reaction

Related factor: Patient's biopsychosocial response to event.

Definition: The stress response pattern that occurs as a result of forcible or attempted forcible sexual penetration against the victim's will and consent. It includes an acute phase of disorganization of the victim's life-style and a long-term process of reorganization of life-style. In the silent reaction, the rape/attempted rape is not verbalized (adapted from NANDA).

■ Defining characteristics

Sudden life-style changes
　　Changing residence
　　Taking trips
　　Seeking out family, friends for support
　　Initiating period of celibacy
Severe anxiety during assessment interview
　　Blocking of associations
　　Long periods of silence
　　Minor stuttering
　　Physical distress
Sudden change in relationships
　　Avoidance of close relationships
　　Irritability toward gender of perpetrator
　　Change in sexual behavior/relationships
Frequent, violent nightmares
Suspiciousness
Persistently low self-confidence and self-esteem
Sudden onset of phobic reactions

■ Suggested alternative diagnoses

None

■ Patient outcomes

Patient acknowledges rape/attempted rape.
Patient verbalizes feelings associated with rape/attempted rape.
Patient verbalizes details of the rape/attempted rape as a means of catharsis.
Patient's stress response symptoms are decreased.
Patient describes a plan that includes safety measures to reduce future risk.
Patient returns to previous level of biopsychosocial functioning.
Other outcomes specific to patient (specify).

■ Target date	■ Documentation interval
Specify estimated date of completion.	Specify frequency.

■ Nursing interventions

Establish therapeutic relationship that will allow exploration of silent reaction.

Confirm with patient that a traumatic event recently occurred, and specifically identify it as "rape."

Explain to patient a rape victim's expected thoughts, feelings, behaviors.

Encourage patient to ventilate own thoughts, feelings, behaviors.

Support and educate significant others. Encourage expression of feelings, and discuss therapeutic response to victim and changed behaviors.

Assist patient/family to establish support network.

Refer patient/family to rape crisis counseling.

Other interventions specific to patient (specify).

Relocation Stress Syndrome

Related factors: Past, concurrent, and recent losses, Losses involved with decision to move, Feeling of powerlessness, Lack of adequate support system, Little or no preparation for the impending move, Moderate to high degree of environmental change, History and types of previous transfers, Impaired psychosocial health status, Decreased physical health status.

Definition: Physiological and/or psychosocial disturbances as a result of transfer from one environment to another (NANDA).

■ **Defining characteristics**

Major	*Minor*
Change in environment/location	Verbalization of unwillingness to relocate
Anxiety	Sleep disturbance
Apprehension	Change in eating habits
Increased confusion (elderly population)	Dependency
Depression	Gastrointestinal disturbances
Loneliness	Increased verbalization of needs
	Insecurity
	Lack of trust
	Restlessness
	Sad affect
	Unfavorable comparison of post/pre-transfer staff
	Verbalization of being concerned/upset about transfer
	Vigilance
	Weight change
	Withdrawal

■ **Suggested alternative diagnoses**

None

■ **Patient outcomes**

Patient demonstrates decrease in physiological/psychosocial disturbances.
Patient demonstrates ability to adjust to new environment.
Patient verbalizes acceptance of new environment.
Patient/family reestablishes a new supportive social network.
Other outcomes specific to patient (specify).

■ **Target date**	■ **Documentation interval**
Specify estimated date of completion.	Specify frequency.

Nursing interventions

Assess patient's orientation, mood (depressed, angry, anxious), and physiological status on admission and q _____.

Assess patient's response to past relocations by interviewing patient and family.

Encourage patient to verbalize thoughts and feelings about relocation.

Establish new environment as close to previous environment as possible to maintain consistency in placement of personal belongings, placement of furniture, pictures, etc.

Involve patient in decision making about care routine.

Orient patient to new environment q _____.

To ease the transfer, encourage family to stay with patient, bring familiar objects from home, and provide familiar socialization.

Encourage verbalization of concerns, feelings, fears about recent change in environment.

Allow patient as much control over his/her situation as possible.

Explore with patient/family methods to expand/develop patient's social network.

Maintain consistency in caregivers and care routines as much as possible. Consider a case manager.

If future transfers are necessary, avoid transfers at night, at change-of-shift, and unplanned or abrupt transfers.

Utilize other resources to assist in transition to new environment.

Other interventions specific to patient (specify).

Role Performance, Altered

Related factors: Surgery, Situational crisis (specify), Psychologic impairment (specify), Chronic illness, Chronic pain, Treatment side effects, Assumption of new role, Unmet expectations for pregnancy, Unmet expectations for childbirth, Others specific to patient (specify).

Definition: Alteration in one's ability to perform those functions and activities expected of a particular role in a given society.

■ Defining characteristics

Concern regarding ability to continue role performance
Denial of role
Conflict in roles
Change in usual patterns of responsibility
Change in physical capacity to resume role
Lack of knowledge of role
Change in self-perception of role
Change in others' perception of role

■ Suggested alternative diagnoses

Caregiver Role Strain (Actual/High Risk)
Parental Role Conflict
Self-Esteem Disturbance
Self-Esteem, Low: Situational

■ Patient outcomes

Patient identifies personal strengths.
Patient acknowledges impact of situation on existing personal relationships/life-style/role performance.
Patient maintains close personal relationships.
Patient demonstrates ability to function within limitations.
Patient verbalizes willingness to consider life-style change.
Patient expresses willingness to use suggested resources on discharge.
Patient describes actual change in function.
Other outcomes specific to patient (specify).

■ Target date ■ Documentation interval

Specify estimated date of completion.   Specify frequency.

■ Nursing interventions

Encourage patient to verbalize consequences of physical and emotional changes that have influenced self-concept.

Encourage patient to verbalize concerns about close personal relationships.

Actively listen to patient/family, and acknowledge reality of concerns about treatments, progress, and prognosis.

Encourage patient/family to air feelings and to grieve.

Provide care in a nonjudgmental manner, maintaining the patient's privacy and dignity.

Assist patient in identifying personal strengths.

Discuss with patient/family the impact of patient's change in role performance and the potential change in family members' role functions.

Help patient identify alternative behaviors that are congruent with a change in personal relationships, life-style, and/or role performance.

Develop a plan of care with patient/family that identifies coping mechanisms and personal strengths and acknowledges limitations. Specify plan.

Assess need for assistance from social services department for planning care with patient/family.

Offer to make initial phone call to appropriate community resources for patient/family.

Other interventions specific to patient (specify).

Self-Care Deficit: Bathing/Hygiene, Dressing/ Grooming, Feeding, Toileting (specify)

Related factors: Depression, Severe anxiety, Developmental disability, Psychologic impairment (specify), Pain/discomfort, Intolerance to activity, Decreased strength and endurance, Neuromuscular impairment, Musculoskeletal impairment, Medically imposed restrictions, Others specific to patient (specify).

Definition: A state in which the individual experiences an impaired ability to perform or complete bathing, hygiene, dressing and grooming, feeding, and toileting activities for oneself (NANDA).

Definitions and descriptors for functional level

	TOTALLY DEPENDENT	MODERATELY DEPENDENT	SEMIDEPENDENT
Bathing	Patient needs complete bath; cannot assist at all.	Nurse supplies all equipment; positions patient; washes back, legs, perineum, and all other parts, as needed. Patient can assist.	Nurse provides all equipment; positions patient in bed/bathroom. Patient completes bath, except for back and feet.
Oral hygiene	Nurse completes entire procedure.	Nurse prepares brush; rinses patient's mouth; positions patient.	Nurse provides equipment; patient does task.
Dressing/ grooming	Patient needs to be dressed and cannot assist the nurse; nurse combs patient's hair.	Nurse combs patient's hair; assists with dressing; buttons and zips clothing, ties shoes.	Nurse gathers items for patient; may button, zip, or tie clothing. Patient dresses self.
Feeding	Patient needs to be fed.	Nurse cuts food; opens containers; positions patient; monitors and encourages eating.	Nurse positions patient; gathers supplies; monitors eating.
Toileting	Patient is incontinent; nurse places patient on bedpan or commode.	Nurse provides bedpan; positions patient on or off bedpan; places patient on bedside commode.	Patient can walk to bathroom/commode with assistance.

■ **Defining characteristics**

Major	*Minor*
Inability to wash body or body parts	Inability to regulate water temperature or flow
Impaired ability to put on or take off necessary items of clothing	Inability to obtain or get to water source
Inability to get to toilet or commode	Impaired ability to obtain or replace articles of clothing
Inability to sit on or rise from toilet or commode	Impaired ability to fasten clothing
Inability to manipulate clothing for toileting	Inability to maintain appearance at a satisfactory level
Inability to carry out proper toilet hygiene	

■ **Suggested alternative diagnoses**

None

■ **Patient outcomes**

Patient is able to perform independent self-care activities.
Patient participates in self-care to optimal level.
Patient acknowledges need for total care.
Patient accepts total care by caregiver.
Other outcomes specific to patient (specify).

■ **Target date**   ■ **Documentation interval**

Specify estimated date of completion.   Specify frequency.

■ **Nursing interventions**

Specify functional level and provide basic care needs as follows:
  Bathing/hygiene ___   Feeding ___
  Dressing/grooming ___   Toileting ___
Discuss limitations in self-care with patient.
Include patient in determining care routine.
Offer pain medications prior to care.
Include family in provision of care.
Use OT/PT as resource in planning patient care activities.
Create opportunities for small successes. Specify.
Acknowledge and reinforce patient's accomplishments.
Encourage independence in performance of self-care, assisting patient only as necessary.
Encourage patient to set own pace during self-care.
Instruct patient in alternative methods for self-care. Specify method and teaching plan: ___.
Plan for postdischarge care with patient and family.
Refer patient and family to social services.
Other interventions specific to patient (specify).

Self-Esteem Disturbance

Related factors: Situational crisis (specify), Psychologic impairment (specify), Chronic illness, Chronic pain, Congenital anomalies, Assumption of new role, Unmet expectations for pregnancy, Unmet expectations for childbirth, Unmet expectations for child, Others specific to patient (specify).

Definition: Negative self-evaluation/feelings about self or self-capabilities, which may be directly or indirectly expressed (NANDA).

■ **Defining characteristics**

Grandiosity
Difficulty in accepting positive feedback; exaggeration of negative feedback
Describes change in social involvement
Verbalization of negative feelings about self
Expressions of shame/guilt
Hypersensitivity to slight or criticism
Nonparticipation in therapy
Lack of eye contact
Lack of follow-through
Difficulty in making decisions
Evaluation of self as unable to deal with events
Hesitation to try new things/situations
Denial of problems obvious to others
Rationalization of personal failures

■ **Suggested alternative diagnoses**

Body Image Disturbance
Role Performance, Altered
Self-Esteem, Low: Chronic
Self-Esteem, Low: Situational

■ **Patient outcomes**

Patient identifies personal strengths.
Patient acknowledges impact of situation on existing personal relationships/life-style/ role performance.
Patient maintains close personal relationships.
Patient verbalizes willingness to consider life-style change.
Patient expresses willingness to use suggested resources on discharge.
Other outcomes specific to patient (specify).

■ **Target date**   ■ **Documentation interval**

Specify estimated date of completion.   Specify frequency.

■ **Nursing interventions**

Encourage patient to verbalize consequences of physical and emotional changes that have influenced self-concept.

Encourage patient to maintain usual daily grooming routine.

Encourage patient to wear clothing to enhance physical and emotional self-esteem.

Encourage patient to verbalize concerns about close personal relationships.

Actively listen to patient/family, and acknowledge reality of concerns about treatments, progress, and prognosis.

Encourage patient/family to air feelings and to grieve.

Provide care in a nonjudgmental manner, maintaining the patient's privacy and dignity.

Assist patient in identifying personal strengths.

Help patient identify alternative behaviors that are congruent with a change in personal relationships, life-style, and/or role performance.

Develop a plan of care with patient/family that identifies coping mechanisms and personal strengths and acknowledges limitations. Specify plan.

Assess need for assistance from social services department for planning care with patient/family.

Offer to make initial phone call to appropriate community resources for patient/family.

Other interventions specific to patient (specify).

Self-Esteem, Low: Chronic

Related factors: Chronic illness, Congenital anomaly, Psychologic impairment (specify), Repeatedly unmet expectations.

Definition: Long-standing, negative self-evaluation/feelings about self or self-capabilities (NANDA).

■ **Defining characteristics**

Major	*Minor*
Consistent verbalization of negative feelings about self	History of lack of success in work or personal life
Consistently expressed feelings of shame/guilt	History of acquiescence to the opinion of others
Expressed inability to deal with events	Lack of eye contact
Rejection of positive feedback	Excessive passivity
Exaggeration of negative feedback about self	Indecisiveness
Reluctance to try new states/things/situations	Excessive seeking of reassurance
	Projection of blame/responsibility for problems
	Excessive positive self-appraisal/bragging
	Self-neglect
	Self-destructive behavior (alcohol, drug abuse)

■ **Suggested alternative diagnoses**

Coping, Ineffective Individual
Hopelessness
Powerlessness
Self-Esteem Disturbance
Self-Esteem, Low: Situational
Thought Processes, Altered

■ **Patient outcomes**

Patient acknowledges personal strengths.
Patient decreases verbalization of low self-esteem.
Patient participates in making decisions regarding plan of care.
Patient practices behaviors that generate self-confidence.
Patient expresses a willingness to seek counseling.
Other outcomes specific to patient (specify).

■ **Target date**	■ **Documentation interval**
Specify estimated date of completion.	Specify frequency.

■ Nursing interventions

Seek assistance from hospital resources as needed (social workers, psychiatric clinical specialist, pastoral care services).

Actively involve patient in developing a plan of care. Plan may include:

Assigning a primary nurse to maintain consistency for patient and to communicate plan to team members.

Assisting patient to identify personal strengths.

Decreasing patient's expression of low self-esteem by:

Redirecting patient's focus to personal strengths.

Giving specific feedback regarding observed positive behaviors.

Setting limits about negative verbalization (frequency, content, audience).

Involving patient in diversional activity.

Encouraging behaviors that increase self-confidence:

Identifying positive coping behaviors.

Teaching positive behavioral skills through role-play, role model, discussion, and so on.

Providing opportunities for skill practice.

Structuring interactions/activities to minimize potential for failure.

Provide information about the value of counseling and available community resources.

Other interventions specific to patient (specify).

Self-Esteem, Low: Situational

Related factor: Situational crisis (specify).

Definition: Negative self-evaluation/feelings about self which develop in response to a loss or change in an individual who previously had a positive self-evaluation (NANDA).

■ **Defining characteristics**

Major	*Minor*
Verbalization of negative feelings about self	Expressed shame/guilt
Episodic negative self-appraisal	Evaluation of self as unable to handle situations/events
	Difficulty in making decisions
	Self-negating verbalizations

■ **Suggested alternative diagnoses**

Adjustment, Impaired
Body Image Disturbance
Coping, Ineffective Individual
Self-Esteem Disturbance
Self-Esteem, Low: Chronic

■ **Patient outcomes**

Patient verbalizes episodic change/loss.
Patient acknowledges personal strengths.
Patient acknowledges low self-esteem.
Patient practices behaviors that generate self-confidence.
Other outcomes specific to patient (specify).

■ **Target date**	■ **Documentation interval**
Specify estimated date of completion.	Specify frequency.

■ Nursing interventions

Explore recent changes with patient that may have influenced low self-esteem.

Encourage patient to verbalize self-evaluation/feelings about self.

Assist patient in identifying personal strengths.

Develop a plan of care with patient/family to generate self-confidence. Plan may include:

> Assigning a primary nurse to maintain consistency for patient and to communicate plan to team members.
>
> Identifying positive coping behaviors.
>
> Teaching positive behavioral skills through role-play, role model, discussion, and so on.
>
> Providing opportunities for skill practice.
>
> Giving specific positive feedback for desired behaviors.
>
> Seeking assistance from hospital resources as needed (social worker, clinical nurse specialist, pastoral care services).

Refer to appropriate community resources.

Other interventions specific to patient (specify).

Self-Mutilation: High Risk

Risk factors: Inability to cope with increased psychological/physiological tension in a healthy manner, Feelings of depression, rejection, self-hatred, separation anxiety, guilt, and depersonalization, Fluctuating emotions, Command hallucinations, Need for sensory stimuli, Parental emotional deprivation, Dysfunctional family, Drug/alcohol abuse.

Groups at Risk: Clients with Borderline Personality Disorder, especially females 16–25 years of age, Clients in psychotic state—frequently males in young adulthood, Emotionally disturbed and/or battered children, Mentally retarded and autistic children, Clients with a history of self-injury, Clients with Multiple Personality Disorder, Clients with history of physical, emotional, or sexual abuse.

Definition: A state in which an individual is at high risk to perform an act upon the self to injure, not kill, which produces tissue damage and possible tension relief (adapted from NANDA).

■ Suggested alternative diagnosis

Violence, High Risk: Self-Directed or Directed at Others

■ Patient outcomes

Patient does not injure self.
Patient is free from self-injury.
Patient reports increasing ability to control impulses to injure self.
Patient verbalizes feelings rather than acting on feelings to injure self.
Patient verbalizes reduction of command hallucinations and/or delusions.
Patient verbalizes absence of command hallucinations and/or delusions.
Other outcomes specific to patient (specify).

■ Target date   ■ Documentation interval

Specify estimated date of completion.   Specify frequency.

■ Nursing interventions

Provide the least restrictive environment that will provide safety for patient. It may be necessary to gradually decrease restrictions based on patient's self-control.

Provide support and education to family regarding patient status and methods of treatment.

Psychotic patient

Assess patient for history of self-injury: methods used, known triggers, etc.

Encourage patient to describe triggers that led up to self-injury in past.

Observe for behavioral changes from baseline assessment, e.g., increased withdrawal, agitation, etc.

Assess patient for morbid preoccupation with suicide, self-mutilation, hopelessness, worthlessness.

Assess patient for command hallucinations determining content and source, e.g., "Whose voice is it? What is the voice telling you to do? Is the voice telling you to hurt yourself and how? Does the voice have control over you?"

Assess patient for religious and/or persecutory delusions that may lead to self-injury.

Assess patient for somatic delusions that may lead to self-injury, e.g., part of body believed to be diseased, rotten, unnecessary, etc.

Observe patient for a calmness in behavior that abruptly follows a period of agitation. Provide increased safety measures to prevent self-injury.

Remove potentially dangerous items from patient and environment recognizing that it is impossible to have a purely "safe environment." Search patient as needed for potentially harmful items.

Administer psychotropic and/or anti-anxiety medications per physician order.

Use seclusion/restraint to protect patient per physician order.

Monitor intensity of hallucinations/delusions and attempt reality-testing q____, assisting patient to differentiate internal stimuli from outside world.

Use protective devices (e.g., mitts, helmet, jacket restraint, long-sleeved shirt, etc.). Obtain physician order if intervention is a denial of rights.

Consider trimming patient's fingernails/toenails to prevent scratching self.

Contract with patient to not injure self. Renew contract q_____.

Encourage patient to verbalize thoughts and impulses vs. storing up tension.

Encourage physical activity.

If patient unable to contract or follow direction, stay with patient at all times until either patient reports a decrease in command hallucinations, delusions, or self-mutilative impulses, or seclusion/restraint is used.

Other interventions specific to patient (specify).

Personality disorder patient

Assess patient for history of self-injury: methods used, known triggers, etc.

Assess patient's level of impulsivity and frustration tolerance.

Encourage patient to seek out staff and peers, not use alcohol or drugs.

Contract with patient to not harm self and to talk with staff about self-injury thoughts or impulses as they occur.

Establish regular and frequent check-in times with assigned staff.

Consider anti-anxiety or neuroleptic medications per physician order.

Provide patient safety with least restrictive measures, e.g., environmental manipulation (removal of harmful objects as feasible, roommate, room close to nursing station, etc.), family/visitor restriction, patient within eyesight at all times, patient within arm's length, seclusion/restraint with physician order.

Provide consistent responses to patient by collaborating closely with other health care providers. Review treatment plan frequently to prevent staff splitting and conflict regarding treatment goals.

Teach patient alternative stress/tension relieving measures, e.g., relaxation techniques, physical exercise, journal writing, self-affirmations, distracting techniques such as music, TV, conversation, etc.

Other interventions specific to patient (specify).

Retarded/autistic patient

Assess patient for history of self-injury behaviors: methods used, known triggers, etc.

Assess patient's response to environment to determine if there is a stressor that may lead to self-injury.

Alter environmental situations that may produce stress that provoke self-injury behaviors.

Remove positive or negative reinforcement that may induce self-injury behavior (e.g., comforting patient after head-banging, excusing patient from perceived unpleasant tasks, etc.)

Develop behavioral plan that will prevent or decrease incidence of self-injury.

Use protective devices to prevent self-injury (e.g., mitts, helmet, jacket restraint, protective clothing, etc.)

Other interventions specific to patient (specify).

Sensory/Perceptual Alterations: Visual, Auditory, Kinesthetic, Gustatory, Tactile, Olfactory (specify)

Related factors: Alcohol/substance abuse (specify), Electrolyte imbalance, Altered sensory reception, transmission, and/or integration secondary to CVA, brain trauma, increased intracranial pressure, and so on, Sensory deficit (specify), Sensory overload, Altered environmental stimuli, Others specific to patient (specify).

Definition: A state in which an individual experiences a change in the amount or interpretation of incoming stimuli accompanied by an absent, diminished, exaggerated, or distorted response to such stimuli. These altered responses are a change from the individual's usual response to stimuli and are not a result of mental or personality disorders (adapted from NANDA and L. Carpenito[1]).

■ Defining characteristics

Major	*Minor*
Anxiety	Complaints of fatigue
Altered abstraction	Alteration in posture
Altered conceptualization	Change in muscular tension
Change in problem-solving abilities	Inappropriate responses
Reported or measured change in	
sensory acuity	
Change in usual response to stimuli	
Indication of alteration in body image	
Apathy	
Disorientation to person, place, time,	
or situation	
Change in behavior pattern	
Restlessness	
Irritability	
Altered communication pattern	

■ Suggested alternative diagnoses

Peripheral Neurovascular Dysfunction: High Risk
Thought Processes, Altered

■ **Patient outcomes**

Patient demonstrates orientation to environment.
Patient demonstrates improving perception of environment.
Patient is oriented to person, place, time, and situation.
Patient interacts appropriately with the environment.
Patient demonstrates the ability to compensate for sensory deficits by maximizing the use of unimpaired senses.
Other outcomes specific to patient (specify).

■ **Target date**   ■ **Documentation interval**

Specify estimated date of completion.   Specify frequency.

■ **Nursing interventions**

Identify factors that contribute to sensory/perceptual alterations, such as sleep deprivation, chemical dependence, medications, treatments, electrolyte imbalance, and so on.
Assess patient's level of consciousness q ___.
Assess changes in patient's neurologic status q ___, and document.
Orient to person, place, time, and situation with each interaction.
Assess patient's ability to follow directions. Develop a plan for self-care, maximizing abilities and acknowledging limitations. Plan is ___.
Develop a plan that maximizes patient's use of unimpaired senses. Plan is ___.
Reduce number of stimuli to achieve appropriate sensory input (for example, dim lights, provide a private room, limit visitors, establish rest periods for patient).
Increase number of stimuli to achieve appropriate sensory input (for example, increase social interaction, schedule contacts, provide radio, television, clock with large numbers).
Explain reason for, and describe location of, surrounding equipment, furniture, and alarms.
Encourage patient/family to verbalize anxiety.
Reassure patient/family that sensory/perceptual deficit is temporary, whenever appropriate.
Monitor amount of sleep in 24-hour period.
Ensure access to and use of sensory assistive devices, such as hearing aid, glasses.
Other interventions specific to patient (specify).

---

[1]Carpenito, L.J.: *Nursing Diagnosis: Application to Clinical Practice* (Philadelphia: Lippincott, 1983).

Sexual Dysfunction

Related factors: Drugs, Surgery, Pain, Disease, Health-related transitions, Altered body function or structure, Illness/medical treatment, Trauma, Lack of significant other, Lack of privacy, Pregnancy, Recent childbirth, Physical/emotional abuse, Sexual trauma/exploitation, Hormonal changes, Body image disturbance, Impaired relationship, Unrealistic expectations of self and partner, Disturbance in self-esteem, Others specific to patient (specify).

Definition: The state in which an individual experiences a change in sexual function that is viewed as unsatisfying, unrewarding, or inadequate (NANDA).

■ Defining characteristics

Verbalization of problem
Conflicts involving values
Seeking confirmation of desirability
Decreased interest in others
Concern over adequacy in meeting sexual desire of partner
Alteration in orgasm/ejaculation
Impotence
Vaginal dryness
Painful coitus
Change in sexual desire
Phobic avoidance of sexual experience

■ Suggested alternative diagnoses

Body Image Disturbance
Rape-Trauma Syndrome: Silent Reaction
Self-Esteem Disturbance
Sexuality Patterns, Altered

■ Patient outcomes

Patient demonstrates willingness to discuss changes in sexual function.
Patient requests needed information about changes in sexual function.
Patient/partner verbalizes understanding of medically imposed restrictions.
Patient/partner participates in problem solving.
Patient/partner actively participates in counseling.
Other outcomes specific to patient (specify).

■ Target date

Specify estimated date of completion

■ Documentation interval

Specify frequency.

■ Nursing interventions

Encourage verbalization of sexual concerns by utilizing caregivers who have an established rapport with patient and are comfortable discussing patient's sexual concerns. Specify caregiver.

Allow time and privacy to address patient's sexual concerns.

Alert patient/partner to possibility of disinterest in, decreased capacity for, or discomfort during sexual activity.

Inform physician of patient's need for information so that teaching may be reinforced.

Provide written information that patient/partner can use as a resource.

Instruct patient in physical illness and treatment interventions that affect sexual function.

Provide information necessary to enhance sexual function (anticipatory guidance, education materials, stress reduction exercises, sensation-enhancing exercises, prosthetics, implants, focused counseling).

Encourage communication between patient and sexual partner.

Inform patient/partner of need for medically imposed limitations on sexual activity and possible consequences (drug side-effects; normal aspects of aging; postsurgical adjustments, especially after surgery on sexual organs or ostomy; post myocardial infarction).

Encourage continuation of counseling after discharge.

Confer with social services to identify appropriate referral for counseling.

Other interventions specific to patient (specify).

Sexuality Patterns, Altered

Related factors: Knowledge/skill deficit, Lack of privacy, Lack of significant other, Ineffective or absent role models, Conflicts with sexual orientation or variant preferences, Fear of pregnancy or acquiring sexually transmitted disease, Impaired relationship with significant other, Body image disturbance, Disturbance in self-esteem, Others specific to patient (specify).

Definition: The state in which an individual expresses concern regarding his or her sexuality patterns (adapted from NANDA).

■ Defining characteristics

Reported difficulties, limitations, or changes in sexual behaviors or activities

■ Suggested alternative diagnoses

Body Image Disturbance
Rape-Trauma Syndrome: Silent Reaction
Self-Esteem Disturbance
Sexual Dysfunction

■ Patient outcomes

Patient verbalizes feelings about sexual identity.
Patient requests needed information about sexuality.
Patient acknowledges importance of discussing sexual issues with partner.
Patient discusses concerns about sexuality.
Patient/partner actively participates in counseling.
Patient expresses satisfaction with sexuality.
Other outcomes specific to patient (specify).

■ Target date   ■ Documentation interval

Specify estimated date of completion.   Specify frequency.

■ **Nursing interventions**

Explore with patient possible causes of altered sexuality pattern (sexual partner, sexual orientation, physical setting, fear of pregnancy or disease).

Encourage verbalization of sexual concerns by utilizing caregivers who have an established rapport with patient and are comfortable discussing patient's sexual concerns. Specify caregiver.

Allow time and privacy to address patient's sexual concerns.

Inform patient/partner of need for limitations in sexual activity and possible consequences.

Provide written information that patient/partner can use as a resource.

Encourage communication between patient and sexual partner.

Encourage continuation of counseling after discharge.

Confer with social services to identify appropriate referral for counseling.

Other interventions specific to patient (specify).

Skin Integrity, Impaired

Related factors: *External (environmental):* Hyperthermia, Hypothermia, Chemical substance, Mechanical factors (shearing forces, pressure, restraint), Radiation, Physical immobilization, Humidity.

Internal (somatic): Medication, Altered nutritional state (obesity, emaciation), Altered metabolic state, Altered circulation, Altered sensation, Altered pigmentation, Skeletal prominence, Developmental factors, Immunologic deficit, Alterations in skin turgor (change in elasticity).

Definition: A state in which the individual's skin is adversely altered (NANDA).

■ Defining characteristics

Disruption of skin surface
Destruction of skin layers
Invasion of body structures

■ Suggested alternative diagnosis

Tissue Integrity, Impaired

■ Patient outcomes

Patient's skin is healed and intact.
Patient is free of further skin breakdown.
Patient/family demonstrates optimal skin/wound care routine.
Other outcomes specific to patient (specify).

■ Target date	■ Documentation interval
Specify estimated date of completion.	Specify frequency.

■ Nursing interventions

Assess condition of skin over bony prominences for breakdown q2 hours and prn, and document.

Include the following in assessment and documentation of wound/skin breakdown:
Location, dimensions, and depth of wound.
Presence or absence of granulation/epithelialization.
Presence or absence of undermining and/or sinus tract formation.
Presence or absence of necrotic tissue. Describe color, odor, amount.
Presence and character of exudate, including tenacity, color, odor.
Presence or absence of symptoms of local wound infection. Consider: presence or absence of pain on palpation, edema, pruritus, induration, warmth, foul odor, eschar, exudate.
Presence or absence of systemic infection.

Refer to ET nurse for assistance with assessment, staging, treatment and documentation of wound care/skin breakdown.

Include in assessment and treatment measures, pressure-relieving devices such as, static air mattress, low-air loss therapy, air-fluidized therapy, water bed.

Establish local wound care measures, which include removal of eschar and necrotic debris, a moist physiologic environment attainable by a variety of dressings and treatment regimens, and consistency in local wound care to achieve the most advantageous wound healing environment.

Assess topical dressing/treatment measures, which may include moisture vapor permeable dressings, hydrocolloid dressings, hydrophilic dressings, absorbent dressings.

Establish a wound/skin care routine, which may include:
Frequent turning and repositioning of patient.
Keep surrounding tissue free from excess moisture, drainage.
Protect patient from fecal/urinary contamination.
Protect patient from other wound/drain-tube excretions into wound.
Consult dietitian for foods high in proteins, minerals, calories, and vitamins. Maintain adequate hydration.
Consult physician regarding implementation of enteral feedings or parenteral nutrition to increase wound healing potential.
Instruct patient/family in skin-care routine, including signs and symptoms of tissue repair, nutritional enhancements to healing, and reportable signs and symptoms.
Other interventions specific to patient (specify).

Skin Integrity, Impaired: High Risk

Risk factors: *External (environmental):* Hypothermia, Hyperthermia, Chemical substances, Mechanical factors (shearing forces, pressure, restraint), Radiation, Physical immobilization, Excretions/secretions, Humidity.

Internal (somatic): Medication, Altered nutritional state (obesity, emaciation), Altered metabolic state, Altered circulation, Altered sensation, Altered pigmentation, Skeletal prominence, Developmental factors, Alterations in skin turgor (change in elasticity), Psychogenic factors, Immunologic factors.

Definition: A state in which the individual's skin is at risk of being adversely altered (NANDA).

■ Suggested alternative diagnoses

Bowel Incontinence
Infection: High risk
Mobility, Impaired Physical
Nutrition, Altered: Less Than Body Requirements
Urinary Incontinence, Functional

■ Patient outcomes

Patient's skin remains intact.
Patient/family maintains and improves tissue tolerance to pressure in order to prevent injury.
Patient/family demonstrates understanding of risk factors that increase chance of acquiring skin breakdown.
Patient/family demonstrates understanding of prevention of skin breakdown.
Patient/family demonstrates optimal skin-care routine.
Other outcomes specific to patient (specify).

■ Target date
■ Documentation interval

Specify estimated date of completion.

Specify frequency.

■ Nursing interventions

Assess patient for risk factors (e.g., bed/chair confinement, inability to move, loss of bowel/bladder control, poor nutrition, and lowered mental awareness) that may lead to skin breakdown on admission and whenever physical condition changes. Document assessment.

Perform systematic skin inspection on all patients at least qd, paying particular attention to the bony prominences. Document assessment.

For mobility/activity deficit

Bed-bound individuals:

Reposition at least q2 hours.

Use pillows or foam wedges to keep bony prominences from direct contact.

Use devices that totally relieve pressure on the heels.

Avoid positioning directly on the trochanter.

Elevate the head of the bed as little and for as short a time as possible.

Use lifting devices to move, rather than drag, individuals during transfers and position changes.

Place at-risk individuals on a pressure-reducing mattress. **Do not use donut-type devices.**

Use proper positioning, transferring, and turning techniques.

Use lubricants to reduce friction injuries.

Chair-bound individuals

Reposition at least every hour.

Have patient shift weight q15 minutes if able.

Use pressure-reducing devices for seating surfaces. **Do not use donut-type devices.**

Consider postural alignment, distribution of weight, balance and stability, and pressure relief when positioning individuals in chairs or wheelchairs.

Use a written care plan.

Presence of moisture or incontinence

Inspect skin at least once/day.

Individualize bathing schedule. Avoid hot water. Use mild cleansing agent.

Minimize environmental factors such as low humidity and cold air. Use moisturizers for dry skin.

Avoid massage over bony prominences.

Check for diaphoresis.

Minimize skin exposure to moisture.

Check for urinary or fecal incontinence q_____.

Assess need for indwelling or condom catheter.

Assess need for protective barrier ointments/creams.

Cleanse skin at time of soiling.

When moisture cannot be controlled, use underpads or briefs that are absorbent and present a quick-drying surface to the skin.

Presence of nutritional deficit

Investigate factors that compromise an apparently well nourished individual's dietary intake (especially protein or calories) and offer support with eating.

Plan and implement a nutritional support and/or supplementation program.

Compare actual weight to ideal body weight.

Request physician order for serum albumin level, packed cell volume, transferrin levels. When albumin level is low, wound healing is impaired and people have increased susceptibility to breakdown.

Consult dietitian for foods high in protein, minerals, and vitamins.

Refer to ET nurse for assistance with prevention, assessment, and treatment of skin breakdown/wounds.

Other interventions specific to patient (specify).

Panel for the Prediction and Prevention of Pressure Ulcers in Adults. Pressure Ulcers in Adults: Prediction and Prevention. *Clinical Practice Guideline, Number 3.* AHCPR Pub. No. 92-0047. Rockville, MD: Agency for Health-Care Policy and Research, Public Health Service, U.S. Department of Health and Human Services, May, 1992.

EL CAMINO HOSPITAL DISTRICT
WOUND ASSESSMENT TOOL

Pt. Name

ID #

Physician Name

Location

Assess on admission and 1 time weekly. RN to specify specific day Wound Assessment Tool documentation in Basic Care Needs. Circle appropriate site description, identify right (R) or left (L) side and use "X" to mark site on body diagrams:

____ Shoulder   ____ Scapula
____ Thoracic spine   ____ Elbow
____ Hip   ____ Sacrum & Coccyx
____ Trochanter   ____ Ischial Tuberosity
____ Medial knee   ____ Lateral knee
____ Medial ankle   ____ Lateral ankle
____ Heel   ____ Other _____

Item	Assessment	Date	Date	Date	Date
Size	Length x width < 2 cm				
	Length x width 2 - 4 cm				
	Length x width 4.1 - 6 cm				
	Length x width 6.1 - 10 cm				
	Length x width > 10 cm				
Depth	Tissues damaged, but no break in skin surface				
	Superficial, abrasion, blister or shallow crater. Even with, &/or elevated above skin surface (e.g., hyperplasia)				
	Deep crater with or without undermining of adjacent tissue				
	Visualization of tissue layers not possible due to necrosis				
	Supporting structures include tendon, joint capsule				
Edges	Indistinct, diffuse, none clearly visible				
	Distinct, attached & even with wound base, outline visible				
	Well-defined, not attached to wound base				
	Rolled under, thickened, not attached to base				
	Fibrotic, scarred or hyperkeratotic				
Under-mining	Undermining < 2 cm				
	Undermining 2-4 cm involving < 50% wound margins				
	Undermining 2-4 cm involving > 50% wound margins				
	Undermining > 4 cm				
	Tunneling &/or sinus tract formation				
Necrotic Tissue Type	None visible				
	White/grey non-viable tissue, & non-adherent yellow slough				
	Loosely adherent, yellow slough				
	Adherent soft black eschar				
	Firmly adherent, hard black eschar				
Necrotic Tissue Amount	None visible				
	< 25% of wound bed covered				
	25% to 50% of wound covered				
	>50% and < 75% of wound covered				
	75% to 100% of wound covered				

3/92

DESCRIPTIONS AND DEFINITIONS

SIZE: Determine by measuring the longest and the widest aspect of the exposed wound surface in centimeters; multiply length x width.

DEPTH: Partial thickness involves the epidermal and the dermal skin layers. Full thickness involves deeper tissue layers - subcutaneous fat, muscle, tendon, and bone. Pick the depth, thickness, most appropriate to the wound using the descriptions.

EDGES: Use this guide:

Indistinct, diffuse	=	unable to clearly distinguish wound outline.
Attached	=	even or flush with wound base, no sides or walls present; flat.
Not attached	=	sides or walls are present; floor or base of wound is deeper than edge.
Rolled under, thickened	=	soft to firm and flexible to touch.
Hyperkeratosis	=	callous-like tissue formation around wound & at edges.
Fibrotic, scarred	=	hard, rigid to touch

UNDERMINING: Consists of tissue destruction underlying intact skin along wound margins. Assess by inserting a cotton-tipped applicator under the wound edge, advance it as far as it will go without using undue force, raise the tip of the applicator so it may be seen or felt on the surface of the skin, mark the surface with a pen and measure the distance from the mark on the skin to the edge of the wound, and use a transparent, circular measuring guide divided into four pie-shaped quadrants to help determine percent of wound involved.

NECROTIC TISSUE TYPE: Pick the type of necrotic tissue that is predominant in the wound according to color, consistency and adherence using this guide:

White/grey non-viable tissue	=	may appear prior to wound opening; skin surface is white or grey.
Non-adherent, yellow slough	=	thin, mucinous substance; scattered throughout wound bed; easily separated from wound tissue
Loosely adherent yellow slough	=	thick, stringy, clumps of debris; attached to wound tissue.
Adherent, soft, black eschar	=	soggy tissue; strongly attached to tissue in center of wound tissue.
Firmly adherent, hard, black eschar	=	firm, crusty tissue; strongly attached to wound base and edges (like a hard scab).

NECROTIC TISSUE AMOUNT: Use a transparent, circular measuring guide divided into four pie-shaped quadrants to help determine percent of wound involved.

Item	Assessment	Date	Date	Date	Date
Exudate Type	None or bloody Serosanguineous: thin, watery, pale red/pink Serous: thin, watery, clear Purulent: thick, opaque, tan/yellow Foul purulent: thick, opaque, yellow/green with odor				
Exudate Amount	None Scant Small Moderate Large				
Skin Color Surrounding Wound	Pink or normal for ethnic group Bright red &/or blanches to touch White or grey pallor, hypopigmented Dark red or purple &/or non-blanchable Black, hyperpigmented				
Peripheral Tissue Edema	Minimal swelling around wound Non-pitting edema extends < 4 cm around wound Non-pitting edema extends > 4 cm around wound Pitting edema extends < 4 cm around wound Crepitus &/or pitting edema extends > 4 cm				
Peripheral Tissue Induration	Minimal firmness around wound Induration < 2 cm around wound Induration 2-4 cm extending < 50% around wound Induration 2-4 cm extending > 50% around wound Induration > 4 cm				
Granulation Tissue	Skin intact or partial thickness wound Bright, beefy red; covers 75% to 100% of wound &/or overgrowth of tissue Bright, beefy red; covers < 75% & > 25% of wound Pink, &/or dull, dusky red &/or covers ≤ 25% of wound No granulation tissue present				
Epithelialization	100% of wound covered, surface intact 75% to 100% of wound covered &/or epithelial tissue extends > 0.5 cm into wound bed 50% to < 75% of wound covered &/or epithelial tissue extends to < 0.5 cm into wound bed 25% to < 50% of wound covered < 25% of wound covered				
NURSE'S	**INITIALS**				

Initials	Signatures and Status	Initials	Signatures and Status

3095 (3/92)

EXUDATE TYPE: Some dressings interact with wound drainage to produce a gel or liquid, so before assessing exudate, gently cleanse the wound with normal saline or water.
Pick the exudate type that is <u>predominant</u> in the wound according to color and consistency, using this guide:

Bloody	=	thin, bright red
Serosanguinous	=	thin, watery pale red to pink
Serous	=	thin, watery, clear
Purulent	=	thin or thick, opaque tan to yellow
Foul purulent	=	thick, opaque yellow to green with offensive odor

EXUDATE AMOUNT: Use a transparent metric measuring guide with circles divided into 4 (25%) pie-shaped quadrants to determine percent of dressing involved with exudate. Use this guide:

None	=	wound tissues dry.
Scant	=	wound tissues moist; no measurable exudate.
Small	=	wound tissues wet; moisture evenly distributed in wound; drainage involves <25% of dressing.
Moderate	=	wound tissues saturated; drainage involves >25% to <75% of dressing.
Large	=	wound tissues bathed in fluid; drainage freely expressed; may or may not be evenly distributed in wound; drainage involves >75% of dressing.

SKIN COLOR SURROUNDING WOUND: Assess tissues within 4 cm. of wound edge. Dark-skinned persons show the colors "bright red" and "dark red" as a deepening of normal ethnic skin color or a purple hue. As healing occurs in dark-skinned persons, the new skin is pink and may never darken.

PERIPHERAL TISSUE EDEMA: Assess tissues within 4cm. of wound edge. Non-pitting edema appears as skin that is shiny and taut. Identify pitting edema by firmly pressing a finger down into the tissues and waiting for 5 seconds, on release of pressure, tissues fail to resume previous position and an indentation appears. Crepitus is accumulation of air or gas in tissues. Use a transparent measuring guide to determine how far edema extends beyond wound.

PERIPHERAL TISSUE INDURATION: Assess tissues within 4cm. of wound edge. Induration is abnormal firmness of tissues with margins. Assess by gently pinching the tissues. Induration results in an inability to pinch the tissues. Use a transparent measuring guide measuring guide divided into four pie-shaped quadrants to help determine percent of area involved.

GRANULATION TISSUE: Granulation tissue is the growth of small blood vessels and connective tissue to fill in full-thickness wounds. Tissue is healthy when bright, beefy red, shiny and granular with a velvety appearance. Poor vascular supply appears as pale pink or blanched to dull, dusky red color.

EPITHELIALIZATION: Epithelialization is the process of epidermal resurfacing and appears as pink or red skin. In partial thickness wounds it can occur throughout the wound bed as well as from the wound edges. In full thickness wounds it occurs from the edges only. Use a transparent, circular measuring guide divided into 4 pie-shaped quadrants to help determine percent of wound involved and to measure the distance the epithelial tissue extends into the wound.

Adapted with permission from Barbara M. Bates-Jensen, R.N., M.N., C.E.T.N.

Sleep Pattern Disturbance

Related factors: Pain/discomfort, Unfamiliar surroundings, Effect of depressants or stimulants, Anxiety, Inactivity, Emotional state, Psychologic impairment (specify), Sleep deprivation secondary to ___ (specify), Medications (specify), Others specific to patient (specify).

Definition: A state in which the individual experiences a disruption in the amount and/or quality of sleep, which interferes with desired life-style (adapted from NANDA).

■ **Defining characteristics**

Major	Minor
Complaints of difficulty in falling asleep	Irritability
	Mood alterations
Awakening earlier or later than desired	Frequent daytime napping
	Frequent yawning
Complaints of not feeling well rested	Decreased attention span
Interrupted sleep	Nocturia
	Regular use of sedative/hypnotic medications
	Regular use of medications that can change sleep patterns
	Restlessness
	Disorientation
	Lethargy
	Listlessness
	Mild, fleeting nystagmus
	Easy arousal
	Nighttime muscle cramps
	Advanced pregnancy
	Slight hand tremor
	Flat affect
	Newborn at home

■ **Suggested alternative diagnoses**

None

■ **Patient outcomes**

Patient identifies measures that will increase rest/sleep.
Patient reports adequate rest.
Patient will sleep ___ hours per night.
Patient's daytime napping will decrease.
Other outcomes specific to patient (specify).

■ Target date   ■ Documentation interval

Specify estimated date of completion.   Specify frequency.

■ Nursing interventions

Assess and document patient's sleeping pattern.

Assess patient's need for sleeping aids.

Provide comfort measures, such as pain medication, back rub, warm milk, and soft music at hour of sleep and nap time. Specify.

Avoid loud noises and use of overhead lights during nighttime sleep, providing quiet, peaceful environment and minimizing interruptions.

Inform patient of necessary interruptions during hospitalization.

Help patient identify possible underlying causes of sleeplessness, such as fear, unresolved problems, and conflicts.

Plan activities to allow time for sleep/rest, avoid unnecessary procedures during sleep period, and limit visiting during rest periods.

Confer with physician regarding need to revise medication regimen when it interferes with sleep pattern.

Find a compatible roommate for the patient, if possible.

Evaluate need for sleep medication, taking into account necessary activities during nighttime.

Reassure patient that irritability and mood alterations are common consequences of sleep deprivation.

Discourage daytime napping by involving patient in activity.

Develop plan to decrease daytime napping. Plan is ___ (specify).

Other interventions specific to patient (specify).

Social Interaction, Impaired

Related factors: Sociocultural conflict, Developmental disability, Knowledge/skill deficit, Communication barriers, Self-concept disturbance, Limited physical mobility, Therapeutic isolation, Psychologic impairment (specify), Chemical dependence, Absence of significant others/peers, Others specific to patient (specify).

Definition: The state in which an individual participates in an insufficient or excessive quantity or quality of social exchange (NANDA).

■ **Defining characteristics**

Major	*Minor*
Verbalization of discomfort in social situations	Family report of change of style or pattern of interaction
Verbalization of inability to achieve a satisfying sense of belonging	
Demonstrated inability to interact with others	
Dysfunctional interaction with others	

■ **Suggested alternative diagnoses**

Communication, Impaired: Verbal
Social Isolation
Thought Processes, Altered

■ **Patient outcomes**

Patient expresses a desire for social contact with others.
Patient acknowledges the effect of own behavior on social interactions.
Patient demonstrates behaviors that may increase/improve social interactions.
Patient verbalizes a sense of belonging.
Other outcomes specific to patient (specify).

■ **Target date**	■ **Documentation interval**
Specify estimated date of completion.	Specify frequency.

■ Nursing interventions

Assess established pattern of interaction between patient and others.
Confer with other disciplines and patient to establish, implement, and evaluate a plan
to increase/improve the patient's interactions with others. Specify plan.
Include the following in plan:
Identifying specific behavior change.
Assigning scheduled interactions.
Establishing structured quiet time.
Assigning primary nurse.
Identifying tasks that will increase/improve social interactions.
Involving supportive peers in giving feedback to patient on social
interactions.
Establishing evaluation checkpoints.
Mediate between patient and others when patient exhibits negative behavior.
Provide information on community resources that will assist the patient to continue
with increasing social interaction after discharge.
Other interventions specific to patient (specify).

Social Isolation

Related factors: Chemical dependence, Psychologic impairment (specify), Medical condition (specify), Treatment-imposed isolation, Alteration in physical appearance, Life-style changes (specify), Others specific to patient (specify).

Definition: A state in which an individual experiences aloneness, which is perceived as a negative or threatened state imposed by others (adapted from NANDA).

■ Defining characteristics

Major	*Minor*
Expressed feelings of rejection	Expressed anger
Expressed feelings of aloneness imposed by others	Expressed feelings of difference from others
Absence of supportive significant other, family, friends, group	Insecurity in public
	Preoccupation with own thoughts
	Withdrawal
	Display of behavior unacceptable to dominant cultural group
	Sad, dull affect
	Evidence of physical/mental handicap

■ Suggested alternative diagnoses

Coping, Ineffective Individual
Post-Trauma Response
Rape-Trauma Syndrome
Relocation Stress Syndrome
Social Interaction, Impaired
Thought Processes, Altered

■ Patient outcomes

Patient identifies behaviors that produce social isolation.
Patient demonstrates beginning acceptance of own personal characteristics that are perceived to contribute to social isolation.
Patient demonstrates behaviors that may decrease social isolation.
Patient identifies community resources that will assist in decreasing social isolation after discharge.
Other outcomes specific to patient (specify).

■ Target date

Specify estimated date of completion.

■ Documentation interval

Specify frequency.

■ Nursing interventions

Identify with patient those factors that may be contributing to feelings of social isolation.

Assist patient to distinguish reality from perceptions.

Confer with other disciplines to establish, implement, and evaluate a plan to decrease the patient's social isolation with others. Specify plan.

Schedule time with patient for social interaction. Scheduled times are ___.

Reinforce efforts by patient/family/friends to establish interactions.

Reduce stigma of isolation by respecting patient's dignity.

Reduce visitor anxiety by explaining reason for isolation precautions and/or equipment.

Provide information on community resources that may decrease patient's social isolation after discharge (community agencies, social agencies, self-improvement classes, counseling). Specify.

Other interventions specific to patient (specify).

Spiritual Distress

Related factors: Discrepancy between spiritual beliefs and prescribed treatment, Separation from religious/cultural ties, Challenge to belief and value system, Test of spiritual beliefs, Others specific to patient (specify).

Definition: A state in which an individual experiences a disruption in his/her belief and value system that is a usual source of security and strength for the person.

■ Defining characteristics

Major	*Minor*
Expressing concern with meaning of life/death and/or belief system	Asking, "Why did this happen to me?"
	Expressing concern about nonadherence to dietary laws
	Inability to participate in usual spiritual rituals
	Seeking spiritual counseling
	Requesting objects associated with worship
	Questioning existence or fairness of deity
	Questioning moral/ethical implications of therapeutic regimen
	Feelings of hopelessness/abandonment
	Disruption in sleep pattern
	Refusal to accept visits from priest, minister, rabbi, and so on
	Anger toward God

■ Suggested alternative diagnosis

Coping, Ineffective Individual

■ Patient outcomes

Patient expresses acceptance of limited religious/cultural ties.
Patient acknowledges that treatment conflicts with belief system.
Patient acknowledges that illness is a challenge to belief system.
Patient demonstrates coping techniques to deal with spiritual distress.
Patient expresses reconciliation with usual belief system.
Other outcomes specific to patient (specify).

■ Target date	■ Documentation interval
Specify estimated date of completion.	Specify frequency.

■ **Nursing interventions**

Clarify patient's religious needs/conflicts:
> Encourage patient to express thoughts and feelings.
> Encourage patient to talk about conflicts and what may be causing them.
> Explain limitations that hospitalization imposes on religious observances.

Identify supportive/helpful measures:
> Communicate acceptance of and respect for patient's religious beliefs by involving the patient in the planning of care.
> Assist patient to identify objects, sacraments, and services that provide spiritual comfort.

Make immediate changes necessary to accommodate patient's needs:
> Provide privacy and time for patient to observe religious practices.
> Contact denominational representative in community and/or hospital on request of patient/family.
> Encourage patient's family or friends to bring special food.
> Provide religious reading material on patient's request.
> Communicate dietary needs (such as kosher food, vegetarian diet, pork-free diet) to dietitian.

Request spiritual consultation to help patient/family determine posthospitalization needs and community resources for support.

Other interventions specific to patient (specify).

Spontaneous Ventilation, Inability to Sustain

Related factors: Metabolic factors (alkalemia, hypokalemia, hypochloremia, hypophosphatemia, anemia), Respiratory muscle fatigue.

Definition: A state in which the response pattern of decreased energy reserves results in an individual's inability to maintain breathing adequate to support life (NANDA).

■ **Defining characteristics**

Major	*Minor*
Dyspnea	Increased restlessness
Increased metabolic rate	Apprehension
	Increased use of accessory muscles
	Decreased tidal volume
	Increased heart rate
	Decreased PO_2
	Increased PCO_2
	Decreased cooperation
	Decreased PaO_2

■ **Patient outcomes**

Patient has adequate energy level to sustain spontaneous breathing.
Patient demonstrates necessary metabolic and physical energy levels to achieve weaning goals.
Patient maintains adequate energy level during weaning process from ventilator.
Patient receives adequate nutrition prior to, during, and following weaning process.
Other outcomes specific to patient (specify).

■ **Suggested alternative diagnosis**

Dysfunctional Ventilatory Weaning Response (DVWR)

■ **Target date**   ■ **Documentation interval**

Specify estimated date of completion.   Specify frequency.

■ **Nursing interventions**

Assess patient's readiness to wean by considering the following respiratory indicators:
    Arterial blood gases stable with PaO_2 >60 on 40–60% oxygen.
    Vital capacity > 13 ml/Kg ideal body weight.
    Length of time on ventilator.
    Maximum inspiratory force > –30 cm H_2O (normal –80 to –1000) so independent respiration can be initiated.
    Unassisted tidal volume > 5 ml/kg ideal body weight.
    Minute volume (VE) > 5–10 L/minute.
    Cough effectively enough to handle secretions.
Assess patient's readiness to wean by considering the following non-respiratory indicators:
    Stable heart rate and rhythm.
    Electrolytes within normal limits for patient.
    Hemoglobin and hematocrit within normal limits for patient.
    Adequate nutritional status as evidenced by acceptable serum albumin, transferrin, midarm muscle circumference > 15th percentile.
    Tolerable pain or discomfort level.
    Absence of fever and/or infection.
    Normal blood pressure for patient.
    Adequate rest and sleep.
    Improving body strength and endurance.
    Psychological/emotional readiness.
    Absence of constipation, diarrhea, or ileus.
Establish effective methods of communication between patient and others (e.g., writing, blinking eyes, squeezing hand, etc.).
Monitor patient's response to current medications and correlate with weaning goals.
Encourage increase in self-care and evaluate patient's response to higher levels of use of energy.
Discuss weaning process and goals with physician and respiratory therapist, including patient's present and pre-existing medication condition(s).
Establish a trusting relationship that instills patient's confidence in nurse to assist patient with weaning process.
Instruct patient/family in weaning process and goals, which should include:
    Why weaning is necessary.
    How patient may feel as process evolves.
    Participation required by patient.
    What patient can expect from nurse.
    Participation of family.
Initiate weaning process by:
    Understanding the rationale for weaning orders (use of CPAP [Continuous Positive Airway Pressure], SIMV [Synchronized Intermittent Mandatory Ventilation], PSV [Pressure Support Ventilation], MMV [Mandatory Minute Ventilation], or T-piece).
    Explain procedure to patient and family.

Check equipment to make sure it is attached to gas source.

Check tubing for kinks and excessive moisture.

Check that settings are as ordered.

Check for presence of bilateral breath sounds.

Measure and record baseline respiratory rate, heart rate, blood pressure, EKG, rhythm lungs sounds, vital capacity, tidal volume, inspiratory force.

Preoxygenate, hyperinflate, suction, reoxygenate patient prior to weaning.

Stay with patient during weaning time to provide coaching and reassurance.

Provide diversions such as television or radio.

Provide a quiet environment during weaning time.

Sit patient in an upright position to decrease abdominal pressure on the diaphragm, allowing for better lung expansion.

Start the weaning time when patient has rest and is awake and alert.

Check vital signs and patient for indicators of non-tolerance or fatigue q5–15 minutes. Reconnect patient to ventilator at pre-weaning setting if indicators of non-tolerance occurs.

Document weaning process and patient's tolerance in nurses notes or flow sheet.

Document in nursing care plan those strategies that promote success with weaning process to ensure consistency (e.g., communication method with patient, family participation, coaching methods, etc.).

Reevaluate appropriateness of weaning process with physician if weaning goals are not attainable.

Other interventions specific to patient (specify).

Suffocation: High Risk

Risk factors: *Internal (individual):* Reduced olfactory sensation, Reduced motor abilities, Lack of safety education, Lack of safety precautions, Cognitive or emotional difficulties, Disease or injury process.

External (environmental): Pillow placed in an infant's crib, Propped bottle placed in an infant's crib, Vehicle warming in closed garage, Children playing with plastic bags or inserting small objects into their mouths or noses, Discarded or unused refrigerators or freezers without removed doors, Children left unattended in bathtubs or pools, Household gas leaks, Smoking in bed, Use of fuel-burning heaters not vented to outside, Low-strung clothesline, Pacifier hung around infant's head, Eating large mouthfuls of food, Others specific to patient (specify).

Definition: Accentuated risk of accidental suffocation (inadequate air available for inhalation) (NANDA).

■ **Suggested alternative diagnoses**

None

■ **Patient outcomes**

Patient/family identifies risks that increase possibility of suffocation.
Patient/family identifies appropriate safety factors that protect individual/child from suffocation.
Patient identifies strategies for prevention of suffocation.
Other outcomes specific to patient (specify).

■ **Target date**	■ **Documentation interval**
Specify estimated date of completion.	Specify frequency.

■ **Nursing interventions**

Assess high-risk areas that may lead to injury to patient/family.
Explore strategies to prevent injury.
Provide educational materials related to strategies and countermeasures and to emergency measures.
Provide information on environmental hazards and characteristics (e.g., stairs, windows, cupboard locks, swimming pools, streets, gates).
Provide information on Poison Control Center and exposure to medications and household products.
Refer to educational classes in the community (CPR, first aid, swimming classes).
Other interventions specific to patient (specify).

Swallowing, Impaired

Related factors: Altered sensory reception, transmission, and/or integration, Irritated oropharyngeal cavity, Mechanical obstruction, Neuromuscular impairment, Fatigue, Psychologic impairment (specify), Others specific to patient (specify).

Definition: The state in which an individual has decreased ability to voluntarily pass fluids and/or solids from the mouth to the stomach (NANDA).

■ Defining characteristics

Major	*Minor*
Observed evidence of difficulty in swallowing (e.g., stasis of food in oral cavity, coughing/choking)	Evidence of aspiration

■ Suggested alternative diagnoses

Aspiration: High Risk
Infant Feeding Pattern, Ineffective
Oral Mucous Membrane, Altered

■ Patient outcomes

Patient tolerates food ingestion without aspiration.
Patient demonstrates increasing improvement in swallowing.
Patient identifies emotional/psychologic factors that interfere with swallowing.
Patient eats independently without choking.
Patient/family identifies appropriate diet and feeding routine.
Other outcomes specific to patient (specify).

■ Target date	■ Documentation interval
Specify estimated date of completion.	Specify frequency.

■ **Nursing interventions**

Provide opportunities for patient to discuss fears related to swallowing.
Reassure patient during episodes of choking.
Consult dietitian for development of meal plan to provide food easily swallowed.
Monitor food ingestion q ___.
Have suction catheter available at bedside, and suction during meals as needed.
Place food on unaffected side of mouth to facilitate swallowing.
When feeding patient, use syringe, if necessary, to facilitate swallowing.
Request occupational therapy consultation.
Place patient in semi- or high-Fowler's position when eating.
Provide positive reinforcement for attempts to swallow independently.
Administer pain medication prior to mealtimes to ensure maximal comfort.
Crush medications to facilitate swallowing.
Involve family during ingestion of food/medications to:
    Review signs and symptoms of aspiration and preventive measures.
    Instruct family about feeding techniques and food preparation.
    Evaluate family's comfort level.
    Provide support and reassurance.
Request social service consultation to help the family determine posthospitalization
    needs and identify sources of community support.
Acknowledge patient's feelings of embarrassment regarding impaired swallowing.
    Teach patient adaptive measures that may help reduce embarrassment.
Other interventions specific to patient (specify).

Therapeutic Regimen Management, Ineffective Individual

Related factors: Complexity of health care system, Complexity of therapeutic regimen, Decisional conflict, Economic difficulties, Excessive demands made on individual or family, Family conflict, Family patterns of health care, Inadequate number and types of cues to action, Knowledge deficits, Mistrust of regimen and/or health care personnel, Perceived seriousness, Perceived susceptibility, Perceived barriers, Perceived benefits, Powerlessness, Social support deficits, Others specific to patient (specify).

Definition: A pattern of regulating and integrating into daily living a program for treatment of illness and the sequelae of illness that is unsatisfactory for meeting specific health goals (NANDA).

■ Defining characteristics

Major	*Minor*
Choices of daily living ineffective for meeting the goals of a treatment or prevention program	Acceleration (expected or unexpected) of illness symptoms
	Verbalized desire to manage the treatment of illness and prevention of sequelae
	Verbalized difficulty with regulation/ integration of one or more prescribed regimens for treatment of illness and its effects or prevention of complications
	Verbalized that did not take action to include treatment regimens in daily routines
	Verbalized that did not take action to reduce risk factors for progression of illness and sequelae

■ Suggested alternative diagnoses

Adjustment, Impaired
Decisional Conflict (specify)
Denial, Ineffective
Health Maintenance, Altered
Noncompliance (specify)

■ **Patient outcomes**

Patient identifies obstacles that interfere with adherence to the therapeutic regimen.
Patient develops plan to achieve therapeutic regimen.
Patient follows plan to achieve therapeutic regimen.
Other outcomes specific to patient (specify).

■ **Target date**	■ **Documentation interval**
Specify estimated date of completion.	Specify frequency.

■ **Nursing interventions**

Assist patient to identify situational obstacles that interfere with adherence to therapeutic regimen.
Interview patient/family to determine "problem areas" in integrating treatment regimen into lifestyle.
Assess patient's level of understanding of illness, complications, recommended treatments to determine knowledge deficit.
Assist patient to develop realistic plan of care to achieve adherence to therapeutic regimen. Plan to include:
    Provision of information on illness, complications, recommended treatments.
    Identification of essential treatments.
    Identification of modifications/adaptations in ADLs.
    Identification of what patient/family is willing to do (e.g., dietary changes, exercise modification, sleep pattern changes, medication schedule, treatment schedules, sexual activity modifications, role change).
    Identification of support systems to achieve therapeutic goals.
    Collaboration with other health care providers to determine how to modify therapeutic regimen without jeopardizing patient's health.
Provide coaching and support to motivate patient's continued adherence to therapy.
Offer information on community resources specific to health goals of patient (e.g., support groups).
Other interventions specific to patient (specify).

Thermoregulation, Ineffective

Related factors: Trauma or illness, Immaturity, Aging, Fluctuating environmental temperature.

Definition: The state in which an individual's temperature fluctuates between hypothermia and hyperthermia (NANDA).

■ **Defining characteristics**

Fluctuations in body temperature above or below normal range

■ **Suggested alternative diagnoses**

None

For specific patient outcomes and nursing interventions, refer to these diagnoses:

Body Temperature, Altered: High Risk
Hyperthermia
Hypothermia

Thought Processes, Altered

Related factors: Mental disorder (specify), Personality disorder (specify), Organic mental disorder (specify), Substance abuse, Others specific to patient (specify).

Definition: A state in which an individual experiences an impairment in cognitive operations, such as conscious thought, reality orientation, problem solving, and judgment. These impairments are a result of mental/personality or chronic organic disorders that may be exacerbated by situational crises (adapted from L. Carpenito[1]).

■ Defining characteristics

Fearful thoughts
Hallucinations
Irritability
Memory deficit/problems
Inaccurate interpretation of environment
Distractibility

■ Suggested alternative diagnoses

Communication, Impaired: Verbal
Sensory/Perceptual Alterations: Visual, Auditory, Kinesthetic, Gustatory, Tactile, Olfactory (specify)

■ Patient outcomes

Patient sustains no injury or harm.
Patient demonstrates improved mental status.
Patient is oriented to person, place, and time.
Patient is oriented to situation.
Patient responds appropriately to questions/situation.
Patient demonstrates improved ability to solve problems.
Patient/family identifies community resources for care after discharge.
Other outcomes specific to patient (specify).

■ Target date

Specify estimated date of completion.

■ Documentation interval

Specify frequency.

■ **Nursing interventions**

Assess and document patient's orientation to person, place, time, and situation
   q ___.
Orient patient as needed:
   Call patient by preferred name.
   Tell patient your name.
   Refer to calendar and clock often.
   Remind patient where he/she is.
   Selectively use TV and radio to assist with orientation.
   Keep frequently used items in same location.
   Use familiar items from home provided by family.
Develop plan for ADLs:
   Involve patient in development.
   Post schedule of activities in room; plan is ___ (specify).
   Communicate patient's skill level to other members of the health care team.
Provide simple explanations while providing care to patient.
Provide a safe environment:
   Assist patient with ambulation and activities as needed.
   Apply soft restraints as necessary.
   Provide adequate lighting (night light).
   Leave bed in low position and use siderails.
   Keep frequently used items in same location.
Provide support to patient/family during patient's periods of disorientation.
Provide positive feedback and reinforcement of appropriate behavior.
Establish a plan for patient's discharge:
   Demonstrate reorientation techniques to family.
   Identify community resources.
   Assist family to identify coping skills.
   Involve social services for additional support.
Other interventions specific to patient (specify).

---

[1]Carpenito, L.J.: *Nursing Diagnosis: Application to Clinical Practice* (Philadelphia: Lippincott, 1983).

Tissue Integrity, Impaired

Related factors: Altered circulation, Nutritional deficit/excess, Fluid deficit/excess, Knowledge deficit, Impaired physical mobility, Chemical irritants (body excretions and secretions, medications), Thermal factors (temperature extremes), Mechanical factors (pressure, shear, friction), Radiation (including therapeutic radiation).

Definition: A state in which an individual experiences damage to mucous membranes or to corneal, integumentary, or subcutaneous tissue (NANDA).

■ Defining characteristics

Damaged or destroyed tissue

For specific and nursing interventions, refer to these diagnoses:

Infection: High Risk
Oral Mucous Membrane, Altered
Pain [Acute]
Sensory/Perceptual Alterations: Visual
Skin Integrity, Impaired

Tissue Perfusion, Altered: Peripheral

Related factors: Interruption of arterial flow, Interruption of venous flow, Exchange problems, Hypovolemia, Hypervolemia.

Definition: The state in which an individual experiences a decrease in nutrition and oxygenation at the cellular level due to a deficit in capillary blood supply (NANDA).

■ Defining characteristics

Skin temperature
Cold extremities
Blue or purple skin on dependent extremity
Skin pale when extremity is lifted
Color does not return when leg is lowered
Diminished arterial pulsations
Shiny skin
Lack of lanugo
Round scars covered with atrophied skin
Gangrene
Slow-growing, dry, brittle nails
Claudication
Blood pressure changes in extremities
Bruits
Slow healing of lesions

■ Suggested alternative diagnoses

Skin Integrity, Impaired
Tissue Integrity, Impaired

■ Patient outcomes

Patient reports decreased numbness and tingling in extremity.
Patient reports increased sensation in extremity.
Patient's edema decreases.
Patient reports acceptable level of comfort.
Patient is able to describe plan for care at home.
Other outcomes specific to patient (specify).

■ Target date

Specify estimated date of completion.

■ Documentation interval

Specify frequency.

■ **Nursing interventions**

Assess affected extremity for color, temperature, sensation, movement, and pain; assess rate, rhythm, and volume of peripheral pulses to evaluate circulation to limb.

Correlate daily assessment with baseline, reporting any increase or decrease in circulation to extremities.

Assess and document presence of edema on scale from 1+ to 4+.

Assess effects of medications on tissue perfusion.

Assess need for antiembolus hose.

Instruct patient to inform nurse of presence or absence of numbness or tingling in extremity.

Offer pain medications q ___, and document response to pain medication. Notify physician if pain is unrelieved.

Elevate extremity above heart q ___ to improve venous blood return.

Place extremity in dependent position q ___ to improve arterial blood flow.

Avoid chemical, mechanical, or thermal trauma to involved extremity.

Discourage leg crossing or sitting for long periods to avoid compromising circulation to extremities.

Use foot cradle to avoid pressure of covers on extremities.

Discourage smoking and use of stimulants.

Encourage active/passive range-of-motion exercises to affected extremities q ___.

Instruct patient/family in methods to provide meticulous hygiene to extremities.

Instruct patient/family to avoid extremes of temperature to extremities.

Instruct patient/family in importance of exercise program, correct diet, and adherence to medication regimen.

Consult dietitian for diet instruction.

Instruct patient/family in reportable signs and symptoms that may require notification of physician.

Other interventions specific to patient (specify).

Tissue Perfusion, Altered: Renal, Cerebral, Cardiopulmonary, Gastrointestinal *(specify type)*

Related factors: Interruption of arterial flow, Interruption of venous flow, Exchange problems, Hypovolemia, Hypervolemia, Others specific to patient (specify).

Definition: The state in which an individual experiences a decrease in nutrition and oxygenation at the cellular level due to a deficit in capillary blood supply (NANDA).

■ Defining characteristics

Skin temperature
Cold extremities
Blue or purple skin on dependent extremity
Skin pale when extremity is lifted
Color does not return when leg is lowered
Diminished arterial pulsations
Shiny skin
Lack of lanugo
Round scars covered with atrophied skin
Gangrene
Slow-growing, dry, brittle nails
Claudication
Blood pressure changes in extremities
Bruits
Slow healing of lesions

The authors have chosen not to develop patient outcomes and nursing interventions for these diagnoses, since the outcomes and interventions are medical/surgical treatments. Nursing's role is to monitor and detect changes in the patient's condition, and nursing care may be better directed by the use of other nursing diagnoses. The following list offers the nurse alternative nursing diagnoses that specifically address the results of impaired perfusion of renal, cerebral, cardiopulmonary, and gastrointestinal tissue.

Renal

Fluid Volume Excess

Cerebral

Communication, Impaired: Verbal
Injury: High Risk
Sensory/Perceptual Alterations: All

Cardiopulmonary

Activity Intolerance
Activity Intolerance: High Risk
Breathing Pattern, Ineffective
Cardiac Output, Decreased
Dysfunctional Ventilatory Weaning
 Response (DVWR)
Fatigue
Gas Exchange, Impaired
Spontaneous Ventilation, Inability to
 Sustain

Gastrointestinal

Infection: High Risk
Pain [Acute]

Further work and development are required for the subcomponents: specifically, cerebral, renal, gastrointestinal (NANDA Taxonomy I Revised).

Trauma: High Risk

Risk factors: *Internal (individual):* Weakness, Poor vision, Balancing difficulties, Reduced temperature or tactile sensation, reduced large or small muscle coordination, Reduced hand-eye coordination, Lack of safety education, Lack of safety precautions, Insufficient finances to purchase safety equipment or effect repairs, Cognitive or emotional difficulties, History of previous trauma.

External (environmental): Slippery floors (e.g., wet or highly waxed), Snow or ice collected on stairs, walkways, Unanchored rugs, Bathtub without handgrip or antislip equipment, Use of unsteady ladders or chairs, Entering unlighted rooms, Unsturdy or absent stair rails, Unanchored electrical wires, Litter or liquid spills on floors or stairways, High beds, Children playing without a gate at the top of stairs, Obstructed passageways, Unsafe window protection in homes with young children, Inappropriate call-for-aid mechanisms for bed-resting clients, Pot handles facing toward front of stove, Bathing in very hot water (e.g., unsupervised bathing of young children), Potential igniting gas leaks, Delayed lighting of gas burner or oven, Experimenting with chemicals or gasoline, Unscreened fires or heaters, Wearing plastic apron or flowing clothes around open flame, Children playing with matches, candles, cigarettes, Inadequately stored combustibles or corrosives (e.g., matches, oily rags, lye), Highly flammable children's toys or clothing, Overloaded fuse boxes, Contact with rapidly moving machinery, Industrial belts, or pulleys, Sliding on coarse bed linen or struggling within bed restraints, Faulty electrical plugs, Frayed wires or defective appliances, Contact with acids or alkalis, Playing with fireworks or gunpowder, Contact with intense cold, Overexposure to sun or sun lamps, radiotherapy, Use of cracked dishware or glasses, Knives stored uncovered, Guns or ammunition stored unlocked, Large icicles hanging from roof, Exposure to dangerous machinery, Children playing with sharp-edged toys, Vulnerable client in a high-crime neighborhood, Driving a mechanically unsafe vehicle, Driving after partaking of alcoholic beverage or drugs, Driving at excessive speeds, Driving without necessary visual aids, Children riding in the front seat in car, Smoking in bed or near oxygen, Overloaded electrical outlets, Grease waste collected on stoves, Use of thin or worn pot holders or mitts, Unrestrained babies riding in car, Nonuse or misuse of necessary headgear for motorized cyclists or young children carried on adult bicycles, Unsafe road or road-crossing conditions, Play or work near vehicle pathways (e.g., driveways, laneways, railroad tracks), Nonuse or misuse of seat restraints, Others specific to patient (specify).

Definition: Accentuated risk of accidental tissue injury (e.g., wound, burn, fracture) (NANDA).

■ **Suggested alternative diagnosis**

Injury: High Risk

■ **Patient outcomes**

Patient/family identifies risks that increase susceptibility to injury.
Patient/family identifies appropriate safety factors that protect individual/child from injury.
Patient identifies strategies that prevent injury.
Patient avoids physical injury.
Other outcomes specific to patient (specify).

■ **Target date**	■ **Documentation interval**
Specify estimated date of completion.	Specify frequency.

■ **Nursing interventions**

Assess high risk areas that may lead to injury to patient/family.
Explore strategies to prevent injury.
Instruct patient/family in safety measures specific to high risk area.
Provide educational materials related to strategies and countermeasures.
Provide information on environmental hazards and characteristics (e.g., stairs, windows, cupboard locks, swimming pools, streets, gates).
Provide information on Poison Control Center and exposure to medications and household products.
Refer to educational classes in the community (CPR, first aid, swimming classes).
Other interventions specific to patient (specify).

Unilateral Neglect

Related factors: One-sided blindness, Neurologic illness or trauma, Blindness in half of the field of vision in one or both eyes (hemianopia), Anesthesia of one side of the body (hemianesthesia), Weakness of one side of body (hemiparesis), Paralysis of one side of body (hemiplegia), Real or pretended ignorance of presence of paralysis (anosognosia), Others specific to patient (specify).

Definition: The state in which an individual is perceptually unaware of and inattentive to one side of the body (NANDA).

■ Defining characteristics

Major	*Minor*
Consistent inattention to stimuli on affected side	Inadequate self-care
	Unsafe physical activity
	Failure to look toward affected side
	Leaving food on plate on affected side

■ Suggested alternative diagnoses

None

■ Patient outcomes

Patient acknowledges extent of deficit.
Patient modifies behavior/environment to accommodate deficit.
Patient's safety is maintained.
Patient demonstrates ability to manage ADLs.
Patient demonstrates improving perception of environment.
Other outcomes specific to patient (specify).

■ Target date	■ Documentation interval
Specify estimated date of completion.	Specify frequency.

■ Nursing interventions

Assess the nature and extent of deficit.

Explain and reinforce nature and extent of deficit to patient/family.

Monitor for changes in deficit.

Consult with OT/PT for assistance in developing a plan of care that challenges the affected side. Consider:

Performance of ADLs.

Safety.

Visual, olfactory, and tactile stimulation.

Most effective methods of providing instruction.

Modification of the environment.

If patient does not respond to aggressive treatment, initiate plan of care directed at safety, simplification of tasks, and environmental adaptations. Consider:

Positioning patient so that unaffected side faces activity.

Approaching patient from the unaffected side.

Placing food in patient's visual field.

Placing frequently used items within view and reach.

Include family in plan of care.

Provide information about community resources.

Other interventions specific to patient (specify).

Urinary Elimination, Altered

Related factors: Multiple causality including anatomic obstruction, sensory, motor impairment, urinary tract infection, Others specific to patient (specify).

Definition: The state in which the individual experiences a disturbance in urine elimination (NANDA).

■ Defining characteristics

Dysuria
Frequency
Hesitancy
Incontinence
Nocturia
Retention
Urgency

For specific patient outcomes and nursing interventions, refer to the following diagnoses:

Urinary Incontinence, Functional
Urinary Incontinence, Reflex
Urinary Incontinence, Stress
Urinary Incontinence, Total
Urinary Incontinence, Urge
Urinary Retention

Urinary Incontinence, Functional

Related factors: Impaired physical mobility, Impaired manual dexterity, Cognitive impairment, Disorientation, Environmental barriers, Unfamiliar environment, Others specific to patient (specify).

Definition: The state in which an individual experiences an involuntary, unpredictable passage of urine (NANDA).

■ Defining characteristics

Urge to void or bladder contractions sufficiently strong to result in loss of urine before reaching an appropriate receptacle

■ Suggested alternative diagnoses

None

■ Patient outcomes

Patient recognizes urge to void.
Patient's mobility restrictions will be ameliorated or alleviated.
Patient's ability to manipulate clothing in time for toileting will improve.
Patient's incontinent episodes are less frequent.
Other outcomes specific to patient (specify).

■ Target date	■ Documentation interval
Specify estimated date of completion.	Specify frequency.

■ Nursing interventions

Discuss with patient/family ways to modify environment to reduce number of wetness
   episodes.
Consider:
   Use of assistive devices, e.g., wheelchairs, canes, walkers, non-skid walking
      shoes.
   Remove loose rugs.
   Improve environmental lighting to enhance vision.
   Provide bedside commode, bedpan, hand-held urinal.
   Install raised toilet seat, hand rails.
Consult with physical/occupational therapy for assistance with manual dexterity.
Consider:
   Obtaining clothing that is easily removed.
   Substitute elastic waistbands and Velcro for zippers, buttons, snap devices,
      hooks whenever feasible.
Instruct patient/family in prompted voiding routine based on patients pattern of
   toileting. Frequent reminders to toilet will decrease wetness episodes.
Offer strategies for bladder management during activities away from home.
Instruct patient/family in skin care–hygiene routine to prevent skin breakdown.
Other interventions specific to patient (specify).

Urinary Incontinence, Reflex

Related factors: Neurologic impairment (e.g., spinal cord lesion that interferes with conduction of cerebral messages above the level of the reflex arc), Others specific to patient (specify).

Definition: The state in which an individual experiences an involuntary loss of urine occurring at somewhat predictable intervals when a specific bladder volume is reached (NANDA).

■ **Defining characteristics**

No awareness of bladder filling
No urge to void or feelings of bladder fullness
Uninhibited bladder contraction/spasm at regular intervals

■ **Suggested alternative diagnosis**

Urinary Incontinence, Total

■ **Patient outcomes**

Patient demonstrates appropriate voiding schedule.
Patient demonstrates intermittent self-catheterization procedure.
Patient is free of urinary tract infection.
Patient is free of skin breakdown.
Patient describes plan for care at home.
Other outcomes specific to patient (specify).

■ **Target date**   ■ **Documentation interval**

Specify estimated date of completion.   Specify frequency.

■ **Nursing interventions**

Identify voiding pattern (either voiding after specified intake or voiding after a specified interval).

Assist patient in maintenance of adequate hygiene and skin care routine.

Consider:

Keeping skin dry.

Application of moisture barrier ointment or skin sealant.

Use of collection device.

Instruct patient in reportable signs/symptoms of urinary tract infection (fever, chills, flank pain, hematuria, change in consistency and odor of urine).

Establish a bladder management program:

Attempt a programmed voiding schedule.

Refer to ET nurse for instruction in clean intermittent self-catheterization, approximately q4–6 hours. while awake.

Maintain fluid intake of approximately 2000 cc/day.

Instruct patient in reportable sign/symptoms of autonomic dysreflexia such as severe hypertension, severe headache, diaphoresis above level of injury, tachycardia of sudden onset.

Consider condom catheter collection device with leg bag.

Instruct patient to self-administer drug therapy program, which may include calcium channel blocking drugs, tricyclic antidepressant in combination with antispasmodic drug, and/or alpha sympathomimetic antagonist drugs.

Other interventions specific to patient (specify).

Urinary Incontinence, Stress

Related factors: Degenerative changes in pelvic muscles and structural supports associated with increased age, High intra-abdominal pressure (e.g., obesity, gravid uterus), Incompetent bladder outlet, Overdistention between voidings, Weak pelvic muscles and structural supports, Others specific to patient (specify).

Definition: The state in which an individual experiences a loss of urine of less than 50 ml occurring with increased abdominal pressure (NANDA).

■ **Defining characteristics**

Major	*Minor*
Reported or observed dribbling with increased abdominal pressure	Urinary urgency
	Urinary frequency (more often than every 2 hours)

■ **Suggested alternative diagnosis**

Urinary Incontinence, Urge

■ **Patient outcomes**

Patient describes plan for improved urinary elimination pattern.
Patient demonstrates ability to implement a timed voiding schedule.
Other outcomes specific to patient (specify).

■ **Target date**	■ **Documentation interval**
Specify estimated date of completion.	Specify frequency.

■ **Nursing interventions**

Instruct patient in techniques that strengthen the sphincter and structural supports of the bladder, e.g., pelvic muscle exercises.
Consult with physician regarding use of biofeedback in conjunction with pelvic muscle exercises and electrostimulation therapy. Consider insertion of pessary if surgical correction not possible.
Encourage patient to void on a timed schedule.
Teach patient not to limit fluid intake in order to decrease incontinence.
Instruct patient in hygiene and skin care measures.
Assist patient to identify and choose appropriate urinary containment devices/pads.
Consult with physician regarding surgical or medical management of incontinent episodes.
Instruct patient in self-administration of oral or topical estrogens to ameliorate symptoms.
Other interventions specific to patient (specify).

Urinary Incontinence, Total

Related factors: Neuropathy preventing transmission of reflex indicating bladder fullness, Neurologic dysfunction causing triggering of micturition at unpredictable times, Independent contraction of detrusor reflex due to surgery, trauma, or disease affecting spinal cord nerves, Anatomic (fistula), Others specific to patient (specify).

Definition: The state in which an individual experiences a continuous and unpredictable loss of urine (NANDA).

■ **Defining characteristics**

Major	*Minor*
Constant flow of urine occurring at unpredictable times without distention or uninhibited bladder contractions/spasms	Lack of perineal or bladder-filling awareness
Unsuccessful refractory treatments	Lack of awareness of incontinence
Nocturia	

■ **Suggested alternative diagnoses**

None

■ **Patient outcomes**

Patient is free of urinary tract infection.
Patient maintains adequate skin integrity.
Patient/family describes plan of care for indwelling foley catheter at home.
Other outcomes specific to patient (specify).

■ **Target date**	■ **Documentation interval**
Specify estimated date of completion.	Specify frequency.

■ **Nursing interventions**

Assess patient for presence of fistula (i.e., urethral, vaginal, rectovaginal).

Assess patient for skin breakdown and maintenance of adequate hygiene and skin care routine.

Consider:

    Frequent peri-care.

    Adequate drying of skin.

    Application of moisture barrier.

    Ointment or skin sealant.

Consult physician about use of indwelling catheter.

Instruct patient/family in use of indwelling catheter management at home.

Instruct patient/family in reportable signs/symptoms of urinary tract infection (fever, chills, flank pain, hematuria, change in consistency and odor of urine).

Other interventions specific to patient (specify).

Urinary Incontinence, Urge

Related factors: Decreased bladder capacity (e.g., history of PID, abdominal surgery, indwelling urinary catheter), Irritation of bladder stretch receptors, causing spasm (e.g., bladder infection), Alcohol intake, Caffeine intake, Increased fluid intake, Increased urine concentration, Overdistention of bladder, Others specific to patient (specify).

Definition: The state in which an individual experiences involuntary passage of urine occurring soon after a strong sense of urgency to void (NANDA).

■ **Defining characteristics**

Major	*Minor*
Urinary urgency	Nocturia (urination more than 2 times per night)
Frequency (voiding more often than every 2 hours)	Voiding in small amounts (less than 100 cc) or in large amounts (more than 500 cc)
Bladder contraction/spasm	Inability to reach toilet in time

■ **Suggested alternative diagnosis**

Urinary Incontinence, Stress

■ **Patient outcomes**

Patient describes bladder management program to restore satisfactory urinary elimination pattern.
Patient's incontinent episodes are less frequent.
Other outcomes specific to patient (specify).

■ **Target date**	■ **Documentation interval**
Specify estimated date of completion.	Specify frequency.

■ **Nursing interventions**

Encourage patient to complete a voiding diary for several days to create awareness of voiding patterns.
Implement a bladder management program.
Consider:
    Encourage a timed voiding schedule based on voiding diary.
    Increase intervals between voiding gradually.
    Encourage fluid intake:_____cc for day;_____cc for PMs; _____cc for nights.
    Teach patient not to limit fluid intake in order to decrease incontinence.
    Instruct patient in use of drug therapy.
    Consult with physician regarding antispasmodic/anticholinergic medications.
    Instruct patient in hygiene and skin care measures.
    Assist patient/family to identify and choose appropriate urinary collection/containment devices.
    Instruct patient in techniques that will increase bladder capacity, such as pelvic floor raising when feeling urge to void, and bladder-training schedule that lengthens time between voids.
    Discourage use of bladder irritants, such as caffeine, alcohol, citrus juices, carbonated drinks, cigarette smoke, and certain spicy foods.
    Assist patient to void prior to sleep and encourage nighttime voids to reduce urgency.
    Provide bedpan, bedside commode, urinal nearby to encourage frequent voiding episodes.
Consult with physician regarding medical management, e.g., electro-stimulation therapy, investigation of underlying irritative or inflammatory bladder disorders, and surgical therapy.
Other interventions specific to patient (specify).

Urinary Retention

Related factors: High urethral pressure caused by weak detrusor, Inhibition of reflex arc, Strong sphincter, Blockage, Others specific to patient (specify).

Definition: The state in which an individual experiences incomplete emptying of the bladder (NANDA).

■ **Defining characteristics**

Major	*Minor*
Bladder distention	Sensation of bladder fullness
Small, frequent voiding or absence of urine output	Dribbling
	Residual urine
	Overflow incontinence

■ **Suggested alternative diagnoses**

None

■ **Patient outcomes**

Patient is free of urinary tract infection.

Patient reports a decrease in bladder spasms.

Patient demonstrates reduced retention by voiding at least ___cc each time he/she urinates.

Patient demonstrates bladder evacuation by clean intermittent self-catheterization procedure.

Patient describes plan of care at home.

Other outcomes specific to patient (specify).

■ **Target date**	■ **Documentation interval**
Specify estimated date of completion.	Specify frequency.

■ Nursing interventions

Identify and document patient's bladder evacuation pattern.

Palpate bladder to determine presence of bladder distention q_____.

Instruct patient in reportable signs/symptoms of urinary tract infection (fever, chills, flank pain, hematuria, change in consistency and odor of urine).

Establish a bladder-evacuation training program.

Consider:

Space fluids throughout the day to ensure adequate intake without bladder overdistention. Encourage oral intake of fluids:_____cc for day;_____cc for PMs;___cc for nights.

Implement techniques that may encourage voiding, such as running water in sink, running warm water over hands, having patient inhale oil of peppermint, providing warm blanket to pelvis, Crede's maneuver, timed voiding schedule.

Refer to ET nurse for instruction in clean intermittent self-catherization q4–6 hours while awake.

Insert indwelling catheter for use at home. Instruct in use of leg bag for urinary collection while ambulating.

Other interventions specific to patient (specify).

Violence, High Risk: Self-Directed or Directed at Others

Risk factors: History of physical/mental abuse by others, Manic excitement, Panic states, Organic brain syndrome, Rage reaction, Suicidal ideation, History of suicide attempts, Temporal lobe epilepsy, History of violence, Arrest/conviction pattern, Substance abuse (specify), Paranoid ideation, History of abuse by spouse, Catatonic excitement, Pain states, Toxic reactions to medications, Command hallucinations, Others specific to patient (specify).

Definition: A state in which an individual experiences behaviors that can be physically harmful either to self or others (NANDA).

■ **Suggested alternative diagnosis**

Self-Mutilation: High Risk

■ **Patient outcomes**

Patient does not harm self/others.
Patient verbalizes anger.
Patient reports a decrease in suicidal thoughts.
Patient identifies support systems in the community.
Patient identifies alternative ways to cope with problems.
Patient reports increasing ability to control anger.
Patient demonstrates increasing ability to control impulses to harm self or others.
Patient identifies effective way to express anger in a nondestructive manner.
Other outcomes specific to patient (specify).

■ Target date	■ Documentation interval
Specify estimated date of completion.	Specify frequency.

■ **Nursing interventions**

Identify behaviors that signal impending violence against self and others. Specify.

Confer with physician on use of appropriate restraining measures when necessary to prevent injury to patient and others.

Clarify use of 72-hour hold for evaluation and treatment in psychiatric unit in the event of abuse against self or others.

Reassure patient that you will protect him/her against own suicidal impulses until able to regain control by:

Taking patient's suicidal ideation seriously.

Frequently checking patient.

Removing harmful objects.

Constantly observing patient.

Assess and document patient's potential for suicide q ___.

Institute suicide precautions as needed (such as 24-hour attendant, room close to nurses' station, removal of potentially harmful objects from room).

Identify situations that provoke violence. Specify.

Encourage patient to verbalize anger.

Confer with physician regarding a psychiatric consultation.

Follow hospital/agency policy regarding legal responsibility for reporting abuse to authorities.

Initiate a multidisciplinary patient care conference to develop a plan of care. Plan may include:

Setting limits on patient's behavior; specify limits.

Providing positive feedback when patient adheres to behavior limits.

Discussing with patient/family the role of anger in self-harm.

Helping patient to control anger by anticipating events that may precipitate aggressive episodes.

Encouraging the use of positive coping mechanisms, such as relaxation techniques, exercise; specify.

Encouraging patient to verbalize anger.

Exploring with patient alternative ways of expressing anger.

Other interventions specific to patient (specify).

■ CLINICAL CONDITIONS GUIDE TO NURSING DIAGNOSES

Medical Conditions
Surgical Conditions
Psychiatric Conditions
Antepartum/Postpartum
   Conditions
Newborn Conditions
Pediatric Conditions

Medical Conditions

Abdominal pain
Acquired immune deficiency
    syndrome (AIDS)
Angina/coronary insufficiency
Arthritis
Autoimmune disorders
Blood disorders
Burns
Cancer
Cerebrovascular accident
    (stroke)
Chest injury
Congestive heart failure
Endocrine disorders
Gastrointestinal bleeding
Immobilized patient

Liver disease
Myocardial infarction (chest
    pain, arrhythmias)
Neurologic disorders
Obesity
Pancreatitis
Pericarditis/endocarditis
Pneumonia
Pulmonary edema
Pulmonary embolism
Renal failure, Acute
Renal failure, Chronic
Respiratory disorders, Chronic
Terminal patient
Urologic disorders
Vascular disease

■ ABDOMINAL PAIN

Activity Intolerance
Related factors: Acute pain, Chronic pain, Weakness/fatigue

Breathing Pattern, Ineffective
Related factors: Acute pain, Chronic pain, Decreased energy/fatigue

Constipation
Related factors: Decreased activity, Decreased fluid intake, Dietary changes, Decreased motility, Medications (specify)

Diarrhea
Related factors: Dietary changes, Increased intestinal motility, Impaction, Medications (specify), Excessive alcohol intake

Fluid Volume Deficit
Related factors: Abnormal fluid loss (specify), Inadequate fluid intake, Abnormal blood loss (specify), Excessive continuous consumption of alcohol

Nutrition, Altered: Less Than Body Requirements
Related factors: Loss of appetite, Nausea and vomiting, Chemical dependence, Emotional disorders, Food intolerance

Pain [Acute]
Related factors: Injury, Noxious stimulus

Pain, Chronic
Related factors: Specific to patient

Sleep Pattern Disturbance
Related factors: Pain/discomfort, Anxiety

Urinary Retention
Related factor: Urethral obstruction

■ ACQUIRED IMMUNE DEFICIENCY SYNDROME (AIDS)

Activity Intolerance
Related factors: Imbalance between oxygen supply and demand, Weakness and fatigue

Activity Intolerance: High Risk
Risk factors: Limited mobility, Frail or debilitated state, Depression, Fatigue

Adjustment, Impaired
Related factors: Inadequate support system, Necessity for major life-style/behavior changes

Airway Clearance, Ineffective
Related factors: Decreased energy/fatigue, Tracheobronchial secretions

Body Image Disturbance
Related factor: Chronic illness

Caregiver Role Strain (Actual/High Risk)
Related factors/risk factors: Illness severity of the care receiver, Unpredictable illness course or instability in the care receiver's health, Duration of caregiving required, Inadequate physical environment for providing care, Lack of respite and recreation for caregiver, Complexity/amount of caregiving tasks.

Coping, Ineffective Family: Compromised
Related factors: Inadequate or incorrect information or understanding by family member/close friend, Chronic illness

Coping, Ineffective Family: Disabling
Related factor: Chronically unresolved feelings

Coping, Ineffective Individual
Related factor: Personal vulnerability in a situational crisis (terminal illness)

Decisional Conflict (specify)
Related factors: Lack of experience with decision making, lack of support system, Interference with support system

Diversional Activity Deficit
Related factors: Frequent/lengthy medical treatments, Long-term hospitalization, Prolonged bed rest

Family Processes, Altered
Related factors: Illness/disability of family member, Lack of adequate support system

Fatigue
Related factors: Disease process, Overwhelming psychologic or emotional demands

Fear
Related factors: Powerlessness, Real threat to own well-being

Fluid Volume Deficit
Related factor: Inadequate fluid intake

Fluid Volume Deficit: High Risk
Risk factor: Excessive loss through normal route

Gas Exchange, Impaired
Related factor: Decreased functional lung tissue secondary to *Pneumocystis* pneumonia

Grieving, Anticipatory
Related factor: Impending death of self

Grieving, Dysfunctional
Related factor: Terminal illness

Home Maintenance Management, Impaired
Related factors: Inadequate support systems, Lack of knowledge, Lack of familiarity with community resources

Hopelessness
Related factor: Failing or deteriorating physical condition

Infection: High Risk
Risk factor: Inadequate acquired immunity

Knowledge Deficit
Related factors: Information misinterpretation, Limited exposure to information (specify)

Mobility, Physical, Impaired
Related factor: Decreased strength and endurance

Nutrition, Altered: Less Than Body Requirements
Related factors: Difficulty in swallowing, Loss of appetite

Pain [Acute]
Related factors: Progression of disease process, Terminal stage of disease

Powerlessness
Related factors: Terminal illness, Treatment regimen

Role Performance, Altered
Related factors: Chronic illness, Situational crisis, Treatment side-effects

Self-Care Deficit: Bathing/Hygiene, Dressing/Grooming, Feeding, Toileting (specify)
Related factors: Decreased strength and endurance, Intolerance to activity

Self-Esteem Disturbance
Related factors: Chronic illness, Situational crisis

Skin Integrity, Impaired
Related factors: Altered nutritional state, Skeletal prominence

Skin Integrity, Impaired: High Risk
Related factors: Alterations in nutritional state, Skeletal prominence

Social Interaction, Impaired
Related factors: Self-concept disturbance, Absence of significant other/peers

Social Isolation
Related factors: Fear by others of contracting disease, Medical condition

Spiritual Distress
Related factors: Challenged belief and value system, Test of spiritual beliefs

Thought Processes, Altered
Related factor: Organic mental disorder

Violence, High Risk: Self-Directed
Risk factor: Suicidal ideation

■ ANGINA/CORONARY INSUFFICIENCY

Activity Intolerance
Related factors: Anxiety, Arrhythmias, Acute pain, Weakness/fatigue

Adjustment, Impaired
Related factors: Assault to self-esteem, Necessity for major life-style/behavior change

Anxiety
Related factors: Threat to self-concept, Threat of death, threat to or change in role functioning

Body Image Disturbance
Related factors: Chronic illness, Treatment side-effects

Breathing Pattern, Ineffective
Related factors: Acute pain, Anxiety

Cardiac Output, Decreased
Related factors: Dysfunctional electrical conduction, Drug toxicity, Ventricular ischemia, Ventricular damage, Ventricular restriction

Coping, Ineffective Individual
Related factor: Personal vulnerability to situational crisis (new diagnosis of illness, declining health)

Denial, Ineffective
Related factor: Fear of consequences

Family Processes, Altered
Related factors: Change in family roles, Hospitalization/changes in environment, Illness/disability of family member

Fear
Related factors: Environmental stressors/hospitalization, Powerlessness, Real or imagined threat to well-being

Hopelessness
Related factor: Failing or deteriorating physical condition

Knowledge Deficit (specify)
Related factors: Information misinterpretation, Limited exposure to information, Unreadiness to learn

Mobility, Impaired Physical
Related factor: Medically prescribed limitations

Noncompliance
Related factors: Denial of illness, Negative consequences of treatment regimen, Negative perception of treatment regimen, Perceived benefits of continued illness, Dysfunctional patient/provider relationship

Pain [Acute]
Related factor: Injury

Personal Identity Disturbance
Related factor: Chronic illness

Powerlessness
Related factors: Illness-related regimen, Chronic illness

Role Performance, Altered
Related factors: Chronic illness, Treatment side-effects

Self-Care Deficit: Bathing/Hygiene, Dressing/Grooming, Feeding, Toileting (specify)
Related factors: Depression, Severe anxiety, Pain/discomfort, Intolerance to activity

Self-Esteem Disturbance
Related factor: Chronic illness

Sexual Dysfunction
Related factors: Pain, Illness/medical treatment

Sleep Pattern Disturbance
Related factors: Pain/discomfort, Anxiety, Inactivity

■ ARTHRITIS

Includes but is not limited to rheumatoid arthritis, osteoarthritis, juvenile rheumatoid arthritis, gouty arthritis.

Activity Intolerance
Related factors: Chronic pain, Weakness, Fatigue

Body Image Disturbance
Related factors: Chronic illness, Progression of joint abnormalities

Coping, Ineffective Individual
Related factor: Personal vulnerability in a situational crisis (new diagnosis of illness, declining health)

Family Processes, Altered
Related factors: Change in family roles, Disability of family member, Lack of support system

Fatigue
Related factors: Pain, Overwhelming psychologic or emotional demand

Home Maintenance Management, Impaired
Related factor: Physical impairment

Knowledge Deficit (specify)
Related factor: Limited exposure to information (side-effects of medication, prevention of further injury)

Mobility, Impaired Physical
Related factors: Musculoskeletal impairment, Pain/discomfort

Pain [Acute]
Related factor: Progression of joint abnormalities

Role Performance, Altered
Related factor: Chronic illness

Self-Care Deficit: All
Related factors: Musculoskeletal impairment, Pain/discomfort

■ AUTOIMMUNE DISORDERS

Includes but is not limited to systemic lupus erythematosus (SLE), scleroderma, vasculitis, rheumatic fever, glomerulonephritis, multiple sclerosis.

Activity Intolerance
Related factors: Anxiety, Acute pain, Chronic pain, Weakness/fatigue

Adjustment, Impaired
Related factors: Necessity for major life-style/behavior change

Aspiration: High Risk
Risk factors: Impaired swallowing, Presence of tracheostomy or endotracheal tube

Body Image Disturbance
Related factors: Chronic illness, Chronic pain

Cardiac Output, Decreased
Related factors: Ventricular restriction, Increased ventricular workload

Caregiver Role Strain (Actual/High Risk)
Related factors/risk factors: Illness severity of care receiver, Duration of caregiving required, Lack of respite and recreation for caregiver, Complexity/amount of caregiving tasks.

Constipation
Related factors: Decreased activity, Medications (specify)

Coping, Ineffective Family: Compromised
Related factors: Chronic illness or disability

Coping, Ineffective Individual
Related factor: Personal vulnerability in a situational crisis (declining health)

Denial, Ineffective
Related factor: Fear of consequences

Diversional Activity Deficit
Related factors: Long-term hospitalization, Frequent/lengthy treatments, Forced inactivity

Family Processes, Altered
Related factors: Complex therapies, Change in family roles, Hospitalization/change in environment, Illness/disability of family member

Fear
Related factors: Environmental stressors/hospitalization, Powerlessness, Real or imagined threat to own well-being

Fluid Volume Excess
Related factor: Decreased urine output secondary to sodium retention

Gas Exchange, Impaired
Related factor: Decreased functional lung tissue

Grieving, Anticipatory
Related factors: Potential loss of body function, Potential loss of social role

Grieving, Dysfunctional
Related factors: Actual loss, Terminal illness, Chronic illness

Home Maintenance Management, Impaired
Related factor: Physical impairment

Hopelessness
Related factors: Failing or deteriorating physical condition, Long-term stress

Infection: High Risk
Risk factors: Immunosuppression, Chronic disease, Pharmaceutical agents

Knowledge Deficit
Related factors: Information misinterpretation (disease process and treatment), Limited exposure to information (disease process and treatment)

Mobility, Impaired Physical
Related factors: Pain/discomfort, Medically prescribed limitations, Musculoskeletal impairment, Neuromuscular impairment

Noncompliance
Related factors: Denial of illness, Negative perception of treatment regimen, Perceived benefits of continued illness, Negative consequences of treatment regimen

Nutrition, Altered: Less Than Body Requirements
Related factors: Difficulty in chewing, Difficulty in swallowing, Loss of appetite, Nausea and vomiting

Pain [Acute]
Related factor: Paresthesia

Pain, Chronic
Related factor: Altered body function

Personal Identity Disturbance
Related factor: Chronic illness

Powerlessness
Related factors: Chronic illness, Terminal illness, Treatment regimen

Protection, Altered
Related factor: Corticosteroid therapy

Role Performance, Altered
Related factors: Chronic illness, Chronic pain

Self-Care Deficit: Bathing/Hygiene, Dressing/Grooming, Feeding, Toileting (specify)
Related factors: Decreased strength and endurance, Pain/discomfort, Intolerance to activity, Neuromuscular impairment, Musculoskeletal impairment

Self-Esteem Disturbance
Related factors: Chronic illness, Chronic pain

Sensory/Perceptual Alterations: Visual, Kinesthetic, Tactile
Related factor: Sensory deficit

Skin Integrity, Impaired
Related factors: Altered circulation, Immunologic deficit, Physical immobilization, Medication

Skin Integrity, Impaired: High Risk
Risk factors: Medication, Altered circulation, Physical immobilization, Immunologic deficit

Sleep Pattern Disturbance
Related factors: Pain/discomfort, Anxiety, Inactivity

Social Interaction, Impaired
Related factors: Self-concept disturbance, Limited physical mobility

Urinary Incontinence, Functional
Related factor: Mobility deficits

■ BLOOD DISORDERS

Includes but is not limited to anemias, coagulation disorders.

Activity Intolerance
Related factors: Imbalance between oxygen supply and demand, Acute pain, Weakness/fatigue, Decreased strength and endurance

Family Processes, Altered
Related factors: Hospitalization/change in environment, Illness/disability of family member

Fear
Related factors: Environmental stressors/hospitalization

Injury: High Risk
Risk factors: Abnormal blood profile, Sickle cell, Decreased hemoglobin

Nutrition, Altered: Less Than Body Requirements
Related factor: Loss of appetite

Pain [Acute]
Related factor: Altered body function

Protection, Altered
Related factors: Abnormal clotting, Bleeding

Self-Esteem, Low: Chronic
Related factor: Chronic illness

■ BURNS

Activity Intolerance
Related factors: Anxiety, Acute pain

Aspiration: High Risk
Risk factors: Presence of tracheostomy or endotracheal tube, Tube feeding, Impaired swallowing, Hindered elevation of upper body

Body Image Disturbance
Related factor: Physical impairment

Body Temperature, Altered: High Risk
Risk factor: Dehydration secondary to impairment in skin integrity

Breathing Pattern, Ineffective
Related factor: Pain

Caregiver Role Strain (Actual/High Risk)
Related factors/risk factors: Illness severity of the care receiver; Complexity/amount of caregiving tasks; Lack of respite and recreation for caregiver.

Constipation
Related factors: Decreased activity, Medications (specify)

Coping, Ineffective Individual
Related factor: Personal vulnerability to situational crisis (presence of burns)

Disuse Syndrome: High Risk
Risk factor: Severe pain

Diversional Activity Deficit
Related factors: Long-term hospitalization, Frequent/lengthy treatments

Family Processes, Altered
Related factors: Complex therapies, Hospitalization/change in environment, Illness/disability of family member

Fatigue
Related factors: Pain, Disease process, Overwhelming psychologic or emotional demands

Fear
Related factors: Environmental stressors/hospitalization, Real or imagined threat to own well-being

Fluid Volume Deficit
Related factor: Abnormal fluid loss (specify)

Infection: High Risk
Risk factors: Tissue destruction and increased environmental exposure

Mobility, Physical, Impaired
Related factors: Pain/discomfort, Medically prescribed limitations, Musculoskeletal impairment

Nutrition, Altered: Less Than Body Requirements
Related factors: Difficulty in swallowing, High metabolic state

Pain [Acute]
Related factor: Injury

Powerlessness
Related factors: Treatment regimen, Health care environment

Self-Care Deficit: Bathing/Hygiene, Dressing/Grooming, Feeding, Toileting (specify)
Related factors: Pain/discomfort, Intolerance to activity, Decreased strength and endurance, Musculoskeletal impairment

Sensory/Perceptual Alteration: Visual, Auditory, Kinesthetic, Gustatory, Tactile, Olfactory (specify)
Related factor: Sensory deficit

Skin Integrity, Impaired
Related factors: Burns, Physical immobilization

Sleep Pattern Disturbance
Related factors: Pain/discomfort, Anxiety

■ CANCER

Activity Intolerance
Related factors: Chronic pain, Weakness, Fatigue

Activity Intolerance: High Risk
Risk factors: Pain, Fatigue, Frail or debilitated state

Adjustment, Impaired
Related factors: Necessity for major lifestyle changes, Incomplete grieving

Airway Clearance, Ineffective
Related factors: Tracheobronchial obstruction, Decreased energy/fatigue, Pain

Anxiety
Related factors: Threat of death, Threat to or change in role functioning, Change in health status

Body Image Disturbance
Related factors: Chronic illness, Treatment side-effects

Bowel Incontinence
Related factors: Decreased awareness of need to defecate, Disease process, Loss of sphincter control

Breathing Pattern, Ineffective
Related factors: Medication, Chronic pain, Decreased energy/fatigue

Caregiver Role Strain (Actual/High Risk)
Related factors/risk factors: Illness severity of the care receiver, Unpredicatable illness course or instability in the care receiver's health, Duration of caregiving required, Inadequate physical environment for providing care, Lack of respite and recreation for caregiver, Complexity/amount of caregiving tasks

Constipation
Related factors: Decreased activity, Dietary changes, Medication (specify), Painful defecation

Coping, Ineffective Family: Disabling
Related factor: Chronically unresolved feelings

Coping, Ineffective Individual
Related factors: Personal vulnerability in a maturational crisis (terminal illness in childhood), Personal vulnerability in a situational crisis (terminal illness)

Decisional Conflict
Related factors: Perceived threat to value system, Lack of relevant information, Multiple or divergent sources of information, Lack of support system

Diarrhea
Related factors: Dietary changes, Impaction, Medication (specify), Stress

Disuse Syndrome: High Risk
Risk factors: Severe pain, Altered level of consciousness

Diversional Activity Deficit
Related factors: Frequent/lengthy medical treatments, Forced inactivity, Long-term hospitalization

Family Processes, Altered
Related factors: Change in family roles, Complex therapies, Hospitalization/ change in environment, Illness/disability of family member, Separation of family members

Fatigue
Related factors: Pain, Disease process, Overwhelming psychologic or emotional demands

Fear
Related factors: Real or imagined threat to own well-being, Environmental stressors/hospitalization

Fluid Volume Deficit
Related factors: Inadequate fliud intake, Abnormal fluid loss (specify)

Fluid Volume Deficit: High Risk
Risk factor: Excessive losses through normal routes

Gas Exchange, Impaired
Related factor: Decreased functional lung tissue secondary to tumor mass or fluid accumulation

Grieving, Anticipatory
Related factor: Impending death of self

Grieving, Dysfunctional
Related factor: Terminal illness

Hopelessness
Related factors: Failing or deteriorating physical condition, Long-term stress, Lost spiritual belief

Infection: High Risk
Risk factors: Immunosuppression, Pharmaceutical agents

Knowledge Deficit (specify)
Related factors: Limited exposure to prescribed treatment information (specify), Cognitive limitations of child (specify)

Mobility, Impaired Physical
Related factors: Decreased strength and endurance, Musculoskeletal impairment, Neuromuscular impairment, Medically prescribed limitations, Pain/discomfort

Nutrition, Altered: Less Than Body Requirements
Related factors: Difficulty in swallowing, Nausea/vomiting, Loss of appetite

Oral Mucous Membrane, Altered
Related factors: Chemotherapy, Radiation to head and neck

Pain [Acute]
Related factor: Ongoing tissue destruction

Powerlessness
Related factor: Terminal illness

Role Performance, Altered
Related factors: Chronic pain, Treatment side-effects

Self-Care Deficit: Bathing/Hygiene, Dressing/Grooming, Feeding, Toileting (specify)
Related factors: Developmental disability, Maturational age, Pain/discomfort, Intolerance to activity, Decreased strength and endurance

Sexual Dysfunction
Related factors: Pain, Disease, Illness/ medical treatment

Skin Integrity, Impaired
Related factors: Radiation, Skeletal prominence, Immunologic deficit

Skin Integrity, Impaired: High Risk
Risk factors: Radiation, Skeletal prominence, Immunologic deficit

Sleep Pattern Disturbance
Related factors: Anxiety, Emotional state, Medically induced regimen, Pain/ discomfort

Social Interaction, Impaired
Related factors: Developmental disability, Self-concept disturbance, Therapeutic isolation

Spiritual Distress
Related factors: Test of spiritual beliefs, Challenged belief and value system

Swallowing, Impaired
Related factors: Irritated oropharyngeal cavity, Mechanical obstruction

■ CEREBROVASCULAR ACCIDENT (STROKE)

Activity Intolerance
Related factors: Anxiety, Weakness/fatigue

Airway Clearance, Ineffective
Related factors: Decreased energy and fatigue, Tracheobronchial secretions

Anxiety
Related factors: Change in health status, Change in role functioning, Change in interaction patterns

Aspiration: High Risk
Risk factors: Reduced level of consciousness, Impaired swallowing, Depressed cough and gag reflexes

Body Image Disturbance
Related factor: Chronic illness

Bowel Incontinence
Related factors: Decreased awareness of need to defecate, Loss of sphincter control

Caregiver Role Strain (Actual/High Risk)
Related factors/risk factors: Illness severity of the care receiver, Unpredictable illness course or instability in the care receiver's health, Duration of caregiving required, Inadequate physical environment for providing care, Lack of respite and recreation for caregiver, Complexity/amount of caregiving tasks

Communication, Impaired: Verbal
Related factors: Aphasia, Inability to speak, Inability to speak clearly

Constipation
Related factors: Decreased activity, Medications (specify)

Coping, Ineffective Family: Compromised
Related factors: Temporary family disorganization and role changes, Chronic illness/disability

Coping, Ineffective Individual
Related factor: Personal vulnerability in a situational crisis (declining health)

Diarrhea
Related factor: Impaction

Disuse Syndrome: High Risk
Risk factors: Altered level of consciousness, Paralysis

Family Processes, Altered
Related factors: Hospitalization/change in environment, Illness/disability of family member, Change in family roles

Fatigue
Related factor: Overwhelming psychologic or emotional demands

Fluid Volume Deficit
Related factor: Inadequate fluid intake

Grieving, Dysfunctional
Related factors: Actual loss, Chronic illness

Health Maintenance, Altered
Related factor: Motor/perceptual impairment

Home Maintenance Management, Impaired
Related factors: Home environment obstacles, Inadequate support system, Lack of familiarity with community resources

Hopelessness
Related factor: Failing or deteriorating physical condition

Injury: High Risk
Risk factors: Altered mobility, Sensory dysfunction

Fluid Volume Deficit: High Risk
Risk factor: Deviations affecting access to or intake or absorption of fluids

Knowledge Deficit (specify)
Related factors: Cognitive deficit, Information misinterpretation

Mobility, Impaired Physical
Related factors: Musculoskeletal impairment, Neuromuscular impairment

Nutrition, Altered: Less Than Body Requirements
Related factors: Difficulty in chewing, Difficulty in swallowing, Nausea/vomiting

Powerlessness
Related factor: Treatment regimen

Relocation Stress Syndrome
Related factors: Change in environment/location, Anxiety, Depression, Verbalization of being concerned/upset about transfer.

Role Performance, Altered
Related factor: Chronic illness

Self-Care Deficit: Bathing/Hygiene, Dressing/Grooming, Feeding, Toileting (specify)
Related factors: Neuromuscular impairment, Musculoskeletal impairment, Decreased strength and endurance, Intolerance to activity

Self-Esteem Disturbance
Related factor: Chronic illness

Sensory/Perceptual Alterations: Visual, Auditory, Kinesthetic, Gustatory, Tactile, Olfactory (specify)
Related factors: Altered sensory reception, transmission, and/or integration

Skin Integrity, Impaired: High Risk
Risk factors: Altered sensation, Immobility, Incontinence of stool or urine

Spiritual Distress
Related factors: Challenged belief and value system, Test of spiritual values

Swallowing, Impaired
Related factors: Neuromuscular impairment, Impaired sensory integration

Therapeutic Regimen Management, Ineffective Individual
Related factors: Complexity of therapeutic regimen, Knowledge deficit, Excessive demands made on individual or family, Social support deficits, Decisional conflict

Urinary Incontinence, Functional
Related factors: Cognitive impairment, Mobility deficit

Urinary Incontinence, Total
Related factor: Neurologic dysfunction

■ CHEST INJURY

Includes but is not limited to hemothorax, pneumothorax.

Activity Intolerance
Related factors: Acute pain, Anxiety, Weakness/fatigue

Aspiration: High Rrisk
Risk factor: Presence of tracheostomy or endotracheal tube

Breathing Pattern, Ineffective
Related factors: Acute pain, Anxiety

Coping, Ineffective Individual
Related factors: Personal vulnerability to situational crisis (presence of acute illness)

Dysfunctional Ventilatory Weaning Response (DVWR)
Related factors: Anxiety, History of ventilator dependence > 1 week, Inappropriate pacing of diminshed ventilatory support, Uncontrolled episodic energy demands or problems

Fear
Related factor: Real or imagined threat to own well-being

Fluid Volume Deficit
Related factor: Abnormal fluid loss (specify)

Gas Exchange, Impaired
Related factor: Decreased functional lung tissue

Mobility, Impaired Physical
Related factor: Pain/discomfort

Pain [Acute]
Related factor: Chest injury

Self-Care Deficit: Bathing/Hygiene, Dressing/Grooming, Feeding, Toileting (specify)
Related factor: Pain/discomfort

Sleep Pattern Disturbance
Related factors: Pain/discomfort, Medically induced regimen

■ **CONGESTIVE HEART FAILURE**

Activity Intolerance
Related factors: Weakness/fatigue, Imbalance between oxygen supply and demand

Adjustment, Impaired
Related factor: Necessity for major life-style/behavior change

Cardiac Output, Decreased
Related factors: Dysfunctional electrical conduction, Increased ventricular workload, Ventricular ischemia, Ventricular damage

Family Processes, Altered
Related factors: Hospitalization/change in environment, Illness/disability of family member

Fatigue
Related factor: Disease process

Fear
Related factor: Real or imagined threat to own well-being

Fluid Volume Excess
Related factor: Decreased urine output secondary to heart failure

Gas Exchange, Impaired
Related factor: Decreased pulmonary blood supply secondary to congestive heart failure

Health Maintenance, Altered
Related factors: Lack of social supports, Lack of material resources

Hopelessness
Related factor: Failing or deteriorating physical condition

Knowledge Deficit (specify)
Related factors: Information misinterpretation, Limited exposure to information

Powerlessness
Related factors: Chronic illness, Treatment regimen

Self-Care Deficit: Bathing/Hygiene, Dressing/Grooming, Feeding, Toileting (specify)
Related factors: Decreased strength and endurance, Intolerance to activity

Sleep Pattern Disturbance
Related factors: Anxiety, Medically induced regimen

■ **ENDOCRINE DISORDERS**

Includes but is not limited to Cushing's disease, diabetes mellitus, hyperthyroidism, hypothyroidism, hypoglycemia, pancreatic tumors.

Adjustment, Impaired
Related factors: Necessity for major life-style/behavior changes, Inadequate support systems

Body Image Disturbance
Related factors: Chronic illness, Treatment side-effects

Coping, Ineffective Individual
Related factor: Personal vulnerability in situational crisis

Family Processes, Altered
Related factors: Change in family roles, Hospitalization/change in environment

Fear
Related factor: Real or imagined threat to own well-being

Fluid Volume Deficit
Related factors: Abnormal fluid loss, Inadequate fluid intake, Failure of regulatory mechanisms

Health Maintenance, Altered
Related factors: Lack of material resources, Lack of social supports

Knowledge Deficit (specify)
Related factors: Limited exposure to information, Limited practice of skill, Information misinterpretation

Nutrition, Altered: Less Than Body Requirements
Related factor: Nausea/vomiting

Nutrition, Altered: More Than Body Requirements
Related factor: Increased appetite

Pain [Acute]
Related factor: Injury

Role Performance, Altered
Related factor: Chronic illness, Treatment side-effects

Self-Esteem Disturbance
Related factor: Chronic illness

Sensory/Perceptual Alterations: Visual, Tactile
Related factor: Sensory deficit

Sexual Dysfunction
Related factor: Disease

Skin Integrity, Impaired: High Risk
Risk factors: Altered circulation, Medications

Therapeutic Regimen Management, Ineffective Individual
Related factors: Complexity of therapeutic regimen, Knowledge deficit, Perceived seriousness, Decisional conflict.

Tissue Perfusion, Altered: Peripheral
Related factor: Impaired arterial circulation

■ GASTROINTESTINAL BLEEDING

Includes but is not limited to hematemesis, melena.

Activity Intolerance
Related factor: Weakness/fatigue

Adjustment, Impaired
Related factor: Necessity for major lifestyle/behavior changes secondary to alcoholism

Coping, Ineffective Individual
Related factor: Personal vulnerability to situational crisis (acute illness)

Diarrhea
Related factor: Increased intestinal motility

Fatigue
Related factor: Disease process

Fear
Related factor: Real or imagined threat to own well-being

Fluid Volume Deficit
Related factor: Abnormal fluid loss (specify)

Nutrition, Altered: Less Than Body Requirements
Related factors: Loss of appetite, Nausea/vomiting

Pain [Acute]
Related factor: Injury

Skin Integrity, Impaired: High Risk
Risk factor: Stool incontinence

Sleep Pattern Ddisturbance
Related factors: Pain/discomfort, Sleep deprivation

■ IMMOBILIZED PATIENT

Activity Intolerance
Related factors: Weakness/fatigue, Acute pain, Chronic pain

Aspiration: High Risk
Risk factor: Hindered elevation of upper body

Constipation
Related factor: Decreased activity

Coping, Ineffective Individual
Related factor: Personal vulnerability to a situational crisis (specify)

Disuse Syndrome: High Risk
Risk factors: Paralysis, Mechanical immobilization, Prescribed immobility

Diversional Activity Deficit
Related factor: Prolonged bed rest

Dysreflexia
Related factor: Spinal cord injury T7 or above

Fear
Related factor: Real or imagined threat to own well-being

Infection: High Risk
Risk factors: Broken skin, Environmental exposure to ___ (specify), Trauma

Mobility, Impaired Physical
Related factors: Medically prescribed limitations, Decreased strength and endurance, Pain/discomfort

Noncompliance
Related factor: Dysfunctional patient/provider relationship

Peripheral Neurovascular Dysfunction: High Risk
Risk factor: Immobilization

Powerlessness
Related factor: Treatment regimen

Self-Care Deficit: Bathing/Hygiene, Dressing/Grooming, Feeding, Toileting (specify)
Related factors: Pain/discomfort, Intolerance to activity, Decreased strength and endurance

Skin Integrity, Impaired
Related factors: Physical immobilization, Altered circulation

Skin Integrity, Impaired: High Risk
Risk factors: Physical immobilization, Altered circulation

Sleep Pattern Disturbance
Related factors: Sleep deprivation, Pain/discomfort

Urinary Incontinence, Functional
Related factor: Neurologic impairment

Urinary Incontinence, Stress
Related factor: Overdistention between voidings

Urinary Incontinence, Total
Related factor: Neurologic dysfunction

■ **LIVER DISEASE**

Includes but is not limited to cirrhosis, hepatitis.

Activity Intolerance
Related factor: Weakness and fatigue

Body Image Disturbance
Related factors: Change in appearance, Chronic illness

Coping, Ineffective Individual
Related factor: Personal vulnerability to situational crisis (new diagnosis of illness, declining health)

Diarrhea
Related factors: Dietary changes, Medication (specify), Stress

Family Processes, Altered
Related factors: Change in family roles, Illness/disability of family member

Fatigue
Related factor: Disease process

Fear
Related factor: Real or imagined threat to own well-being

Fluid Volume Deficit
Related factors: Abnormal fluid loss (specify), Inadequate fluid intake

Fluid Volume Excess
Related factors: Malnutrition, Portal hypertension

Knowledge Deficit (specify)
Related factors: Information misinterpretation, Unreadiness to learn

Mobility, Impaired Physical
Related factors: Pain/discomfort, Decreased strength and endurance

Nutrition, Altered: Less Than Body Requirements
Related factors: Loss of appetite, Nausea/vomiting

Pain [Acute]
Related factor: Injury

Role Performance, Altered
Related factor: Chronic illness

Self-Care Deficit: Bathing/Hygiene, Dressing/Grooming, Feeding, Toileting (specify)
Related factors: Pain/discomfort, Intolerance to activity

Self-Esteem Disturbance
Related factors: Chronic illness, Situational crisis

Skin Integrity, Impaired: High Risk
Risk factor: Physical immobilization

Social Interaction, Impaired
Related factor: Chemical dependence

Thought Processes, Altered
Related factors: Chronic organic disorder, Substance abuse

■ MYOCARDIAL INFARCTION (CHEST PAIN, ARRHYTHMIAS)

Activity Intolerance
Related factors: Acute pain, Weakness/fatigue, Arrhythmias

Anxiety
Related factors: Threat to or change in health status, Threat to or change in role functioning

Cardiac Output, Decreased
Related factors: Dysfunctional electrical conduction, Increased ventricular workload, Ventricular ischemia, Ventricular damage

Coping, Ineffective Individual
Related factor: Personal vulnerability to situational crisis (new diagnosis of illness, declining health)

Denial, Ineffective
Related factor: Fear of consequences

Family Processes, Altered
Related factors: Change in family roles, Hospitalization/change in environment

Fatigue
Related factor: Disease process

Fear
Related factor: Real or imagined threat to own well-being

Fluid Volume Excess
Related factor: Decreased urine output secondary to heart failure

Gas Exchange, Impaired
Related factors: Decreased pulmonary blood supply secondary to pulmonary hypertension/congestive heart failure

Health Maintenance, Altered
Related factor: Lack of social supports

Pain [Acute]
Related factor: Myocardial ischemia

Powerlessness
Related factor: Treatment regimen

Role Performance, Altered
Related factors: Situational crisis, Treatment side-effects

Self-Care Deficit: Bathing/Hygiene, Dressing/Grooming, Feeding, Toileting (specify)
Related factors: Pain/discomfort, Intolerance to activity

Self-Esteem Disturbance
Related factor: Treatment side-effects

Sexual Dysfunction
Related factors: Disease, Health-related transitions, Illness/medical treatment

Sleep Pattern Disturbance
Related factors: Sleep deprivation, Pain/discomfort

■ NEUROLOGIC DISORDERS

Includes but is not limited to multiple sclerosis, amyotrophic lateral sclerosis, brain tumors, Guillain-Barré syndrome, myasthenia gravis, seizure disorders, Alzheimer's disease, coma, head injury, cerebral thrombosis, transient ischemic attack.

Associated psychiatric diagnoses: central nervous system infections (tertiary neurosyphilis, viral encephalitis, Jakob-Creutzfeldt disease, etc.), brain trauma, Huntington's chorea, Parkinson's disease, meningitis.

Activity Intolerance
Related factors: Acute pain, Chronic pain, Weakness/fatigue

Adjustment, Impaired
Related factors: Inadequate support systems, Necessity for major life-style/behavior changes

Airway Clearance, Ineffective
Related factor: Decreased energy/fatigue

Anxiety
Related factors: Change in health status, Threat to or change in role functioning, Change in interaction pattern

Aspiration: High Risk
Risk factors: Impaired swallowing, Presence of tracheostomy or endotracheal tube, Reduced level of consciousness, Depressed cough and gag reflexes, Tube feedings, Hindered elevation of upper body

Body Image Disturbance
Related factors: Chronic illness, Surgery, Treatment side-effects

Bowel Incontinence
Related factors: Decreased awareness of need to defecate, Loss of sphincter control

Breathing Pattern, Ineffective
Related factors: Neuromuscular paralysis/weakness, Decreased energy/fatigue

Communication, Impaired: Verbal
Related factors: Psychologic impairment, Aphasia, Inability to speak, Inability to speak clearly, Tracheostomy

Constipation
Related factor: Decreased activity

Coping, Ineffective Family: Compromised
Related factors: Temporary family disorganization and role changes, Chronic illness/disability

Coping, Ineffective Individual
Related factor: Personal vulnerability to situational crisis (new diagnosis of illness, declining health, terminal illness)

Disuse Syndrome: High Risk
Risk factors: Paralysis, Altered level of consciousness

Diversional Activity Deficit
Related factors: Forced inactivity, Long-term hospitalization

Dysfunctional Ventilatory Weaning Response (DVWR)
Related factors: History of ventilator dependence > 1 week, Ineffective airway clearance, Anxiety

Family Processes, Altered
Related factors: Change in family roles, Change in family structure, Illness/disability of family member, Hospitalization/change in environment

Fatigue
Related factor: Disease process

Fear
Related factor: Real threat to well-being

Fluid Volume Deficit
Related factor: Inadequate fluid intake

Fluid Volume Deficit: High Risk
Risk factor: Deviation affecting access to intake or absorption of fluid

Home Maintenance Management, Impaired
Related factors: Home environment obstacles, Inadequate support system, Insufficient family organization or planning, Psychologic impairment, Lack of familiarity with community resources

Hopelessness
Related factor: Failing or deteriorating physical condition

Injury: High Risk
Risk factors: Sensory dysfunction; Orientation, cognitive, affective, and psychomotor factors

Knowledge Deficit (specify)
Related factor: Cognitive limitations

Mobility, Impaired Physical
Related factors: Neuromuscular impairment, Decreased strength and endurance, Pain/discomfort, Medically prescribed treatment

Noncompliance
Related factors: Denial of illness, Negative perception of treatment regimen

Nutrition, Altered: Less Than Body Requirements
Related factors: Difficulty in chewing, Difficulty in swallowing, Psychologic impairment, Loss of appetite

Pain, Chronic
Related factor: Neurologic injury

Powerlessness
Related factor: Chronic illness

Role Performance, Altered
Related factors: Chronic illness, Treatment side-effects

Self-Care Deficit: Bathing/Hygiene, Dressing/Grooming, Feeding, Toileting (specify)
Related factors: Pain/discomfort, Decreased strength and endurance, Neuromuscular impairment, Psychologic impairment

Self-Esteem Disturbance
Related factor: Chronic illness

Sensory/Perceptual Alterations: Visual, Auditory, Kinesthetic, Gustatory, Tactile, Olfactory (specify)
Related factors: Altered sensory reception, transmission, and/or integration, Sensory deficit, Sensory overload

Skin Integrity, Impaired
Related factors: Physical immobilization, Altered circulation

Skin Integrity, Impaired: High Risk
Risk factors: Physical immobilization, Altered circulation

Sleep Pattern Disturbance
Related factor: Psychologic impairment

Social Interaction, Impaired
Related factors: Communication barriers, Self-concept disturbance, Therapeutic isolation

Swallowing, Impaired
Related factors: Neuromuscular impairment, Psychologic impairment, Altered sensory transmission, reception, and/or integration

Thought Processes, Altered
Related factor: Chronic organic disorder

Urinary Incontinence, Functional
Related factors: Cognitive impairment, Mobility deficit, Disorientation

Urinary Incontinence, Total
Related factor: Neurologic dysfunction

Violence, High Risk: Self-Directed or Directed at Others
Risk factor: Organic mental disorder

■ OBESITY

Activity Intolerance
Related factor: Sedentary life-style

Body Image Disturbance
Related factors: Eating disorder, Psychologic impairment

Coping, Ineffective Individual
Related factor: Personal vulnerability in situational crisis

Fatigue
Related factor: Energy requirements to perform activities of daily living

Health Maintenance, Altered
Related factor: Lack of ability to make deliberate and thoughtful judgments

Health-Seeking Behaviors
Related factors: Specific to patient

Mobility, Impaired Physical
Related factor: Decreased strength and endurance

Nutrition, Altered: More Than Body Requirements
Related factors: Eating disorder, Lack of physical exercise, Decreased metabolic requirements, Lack of basic nutritional knowledge

Self-Esteem Disturbance
Related factor: Psychologic impairment

Sexuality Patterns, Altered
Related factor: Body image disturbance

Skin Integrity, Impaired: High Risk
Risk factor: Alterations in nutritional state

Sleep Pattern Disturbance
Related factors: Discomfort, Activity

Social Interaction, Impaired
Related factor: Self-concept disturbance

Therapeutic Regimen Management, Ineffective Individual
Related factors: Decisional conflict, Perceived barriers, Perceived susceptibility, Social support deficits, Family patterns of health care

■ PANCREATITIS

Activity Intolerance
Related factors: Acute pain, Weakness/fatigue

Diarrhea
Related factor: Medication (specify)

Family Processes, Altered
Related factors: Hospitalization/change in environment, Change in family roles

Fatigue
Related factors: Disease process, Pain

Fear
Related factor: Real or imagined threat to own well-being

Fluid Volume Deficit
Related factors: Abnormal fluid loss (specify), Inadequate fluid intake

Health Maintenance, Altered
Related factor: Lack of ability to make deliberate and thoughtful judgments

Noncompliance
Related factors: Negative perception of treatment regimen, Dysfunctional relationship between patient and provider

Nutrition, Altered: Less Than Body Requirements
Related factors: Loss of appetite, Nausea/vomiting, Chemical dependence

Pain [Acute]
Related factor: Injury

Self-Care Deficit: Bathing/Hygiene, Dressing/Grooming, Feeding, Toileting (specify)
Related factors: Pain/discomfort, Intolerance to activity

Self-Esteem Disturbance
Related factor: Chronic illness

Sleep Pattern Disturbance
Related factor: Sleep deprivation

Therapeutic Regimen Management, Ineffective Individual
Related factors: Perceived susceptibility, Family conflict, Mistrust of regimen and/or health care personnel, Decisional conflict

Thought Processes, Altered
Related factor: Substance abuse

■ PERICARDITIS/ENDOCARDITIS

Anxiety
Related factor: Threat to health status

Breathing Pattern, Ineffective
Related factor: Acute pain

Cardiac Output, Decreased
Related factors: Dysfunctional electrical conduction, Increased ventricular workload

Fear
Related factor: Real or imagined threat to own well-being

Pain [Acute]
Related factor: Inflammation

Self-Care Deficit: Bathing/Hygiene, Dressing/Grooming, Feeding, Toileting (specify)
Related factors: Pain/discomfort, Decreased strength and endurance

---

■ PNEUMONIA

Activity Intolerance
Related factors: Weakness/fatigue

Airway Clearance, Ineffective
Related factor: Pain

Anxiety
Related factor: Threat to or change to health status

Fluid Volume Deficit: High Risk
Risk factor: Factors affecting fluid needs

Gas Exchange, Impaired
Related factor: Decreased functional lung tissue secondary to pneumonia

Nutrition, Altered: Less Than Body Requirements
Related factor: Loss of appetite

Pain [Acute]
Related factor: Injury

Self-Care Deficit: Bathing/Hygiene, Dressing/Grooming, Feeding, Toileting (specify)
Related factors: Pain/discomfort, Intolerance to activity

Sleep Pattern Disturbance
Related factor: Sleep deprivation

■ PULMONARY EDEMA

Activity Intolerance
Related factors: Imbalance between oxygen supply and demand, Weakness/fatigue

Cardiac Output, Decreased
Related factor: Increased ventricular workload

Fatigue
Related factor: Disease process

Fear
Related factor: Environmental stressors/hospitalization

Fluid Volume Excess
Related factor: Decreased urine output secondary to pulmonary edema

Nutrition, Altered: Less Than Body Requirements
Related factor: Loss of appetite

Self-Care Deficit: Bathing/Hygiene, Dressing/Grooming, Feeding, Toileting (specify)
Related factors: Pain/discomfort, Intolerance to activity

Sleep Pattern Disturbance
Related factor: Sleep deprivation

■ PULMONARY EMBOLISM

Activity Intolerance
Related factors: Acute pain, Imbalance between oxygen supply and demand

Diversional Activity Deficit
Related factors: Prolonged bed rest, Forced inactivity

Fear
Related factor: Real or imagined threat to own well-being

Gas Exchange, Impaired
Related factor: Decreased pulmonary blood supply secondary to pulmonary embolus

Self-Care Deficit: Bathing/Hygiene, Dressing/Grooming, Feeding, Toileting (specify)
Related factors: Pain/discomfort, Intolerance to activity

■ RENAL FAILURE, ACUTE

Body Image Disturbance
Related factors: Treatment side-effects, Situational crisis

Breathing Pattern, Ineffective
Related factors: Decreased energy/ fatigue, Fluid overload

Cardiac Output, Decreased
Related factor: Increased ventricular workload

Coping, Ineffective Individual
Related factor: Personal vulnerability in situational crisis (new diagnosis of illness)

Denial, Ineffective
Related factor: Fear of consequences

Family Processes, Altered
Related factors: Hospitalization/change in environment, Change in family roles, Illness/disability of family member

Fear
Related factors: Environmental stress-ors/hospitalization, Powerlessness, Real threat to own well-being, Real threat to child

Fluid Volume Excess
Related factors: Increased fluid intake, Decreased urine output

Infection: High Rrisk
Risk factor: Invasive therapy

Nutrition, Altered: Less Than Body Requirements
Related factors: Loss of appetite, Nausea/vomiting, Dietary restrictions

Personal Identity Disturbance
Related factor: Situational crisis

Powerlessness
Related factor: Treatment regimen

Role Performance, Altered
Related factor: Treatment side-effects

Self-Esteem Disturbance
Related factor: Treatment side-effects

Therapeutic Regimen Management, Ineffective Individual
Related factors: Complexity of thera-peutic regimen, Knowledge deficits, Perceived seriousness, Perceived benefits

■ RENAL FAILURE, CHRONIC

Activity Intolerance
Related factor: Weakness/fatigue secondary to anemia

Adjustment, Impaired
Related factors: Assault to self-esteem, Pattern of dependence

Body Image Disturbance
Related factors: Altered growth and development, Treatment side-effects, Chronic illness, Surgery (hemodialysis blood access, peritoneal catheter, amputations)

Breathing Pattern, Ineffective
Related factors: Anemia, Volume overload

Cardiac Output, Decreased
Related factors: Drug toxicity, Increased ventricular workload

Caregiver Role Strain (Actual/High Risk)
Related factors/risk factors: Complexity/ amount of caregiving tasks, Illness severity of the health care receiver, Care receiver exhibits deviant, bizarre behavior, Situational stressors within the family, Chronicity of caregiving, Caregiver's health, knowledge, skills, experience, competing role commit-ments, coping styles, isolation, opportu-nity for respite and recreation

Communication, Impaired: Verbal
Related factor: Acute confusion

Constipation
Related factor: Medication (specify)

Coping, Ineffective Family: Disabling
Related factors: Chronically unresolved feelings, Conflicting coping styles

Coping, Ineffective Individual
Related factors: Personal vulnerability in situational crisis (new diagnosis of chronic illness, declining health, terminal illness)

Denial, Ineffective
Related factor: Fear of consequences

Diversional Activity Deficit
Related factor: Frequent/lengthy medical treatments

Family Processes, Altered
Related factor: Illness/disability of family member

Fatigue
Related factor: Overwhelming psychologic or emotional demands

Fear
Related factors: Environmental stressors/hospitalization, Powerlessness, Real or imagined threat to well-being

Fluid Volume Deficit
Related factors: Abnormal fluid loss (specify), Abnormal blood loss secondary to hemodialysis procedure, Inadequate fluid intake

Fluid Volume Excess
Related factors: Increased fluid intake secondary to excess sodium intake, sodium retention, Hyperglycemia, Noncompliance with fluid restriction

Grieving, Dysfunctional
Related factors: Chronic illness, Loss, Terminal illness

Health Maintenance, Altered
Related factors: Lack of social supports, Lack of material resources

Hopelessness
Related factors: Failing or deteriorating physical condition, Lack of social supports, Long-term stress

Infection: High Risk
Risk factors: Immunosuppression, Malnutrition, Invasive therapy

Injury: High Risk
Risk factors: Altered mobility, Sensory dysfunction, Hypotension, Weakness

Knowledge Deficit (specify)
Related factors: Limited understanding of prescribed treatment, Limited practice of skill (specify)

Mobility, Impaired Physical
Related factors: Decreased strength and endurance secondary to anemia, Musculoskeletal impairment, Neuromuscular impairment

Noncompliance
Related factors: Denial of illness, Dysfunctional relationship between patient and provider, Negative consequence of treatment regimen, Negative perception of treatment regimen, Perceived benefits of continued illness

Nutrition, Altered: Less Than Body Requirements
Related factors: Loss of appetite, Nausea/vomiting

Pain [Acute]
Related factors: Paresthesia, Muscle cramps, Pruritus

Powerlessness
Related factors: Treatment regimen, Chronic illness

Role Performance, Altered
Related factors: Chronic illness, Treatment side-effects

Self-Care Deficit: Bathing/Hygiene, Dressing/Grooming, Feeding, Toileting (specify)
Related factors: Depression, Pain/discomfort, Intolerance to activity, Decreased strength and endurance, Neuromuscular impairment, Musculoskeletal impairment

Self-Esteem Disturbance
Related factors: Altered growth and development, Chronic illness, Surgery (hemodialysis blood access, peritoneal catheter, amputations), Treatment side-effects

Sensory/Perceptual Alterations: Visual, Kinesthetic, Gustatory, Tactile (specify)
Related factor: Sensory deficit secondary to diabetic retinopathy, peripheral neuropathy

Sexual Dysfunction
Related factors: Disturbance in self-esteem, Impotence, Loss of libido

Skin Integrity, Impaired: High Rrisk
Risk factors: Alterations in nutritional state, Altered circulation

Sleep Pattern Disturbance
Related factor: Sleep deprivation secondary to insomnia

Social Isolation
Related factors: Medical condition, Alteration in physical appearance, Lifestyle changes

Therapeutic Regimen Management, Ineffective Individual
Related factors: Complexity of therapeutic regimen, Knowledge deficits, Perceived seriousness, Perceived benefits

Tissue Perfusion, Altered: Peripheral
Related factors: Impaired venous circulation secondary to surgical creation of hemodialysis blood access, Impaired arterial circulation secondary to hypertension, Diabetes

■ RESPIRATORY DISORDERS, CHRONIC

Includes but is not limited to asthma, chronic obstructive pulmonary disease, chronic restrictive pulmonary disease.

Activity Intolerance
Related factors: Weakness/fatigue, Imbalance between oxygen supply and demand, Anxiety

Adjustment, Impaired
Related factors: Necessity for major lifestyle/behavior change secondary to chronic illness, Pattern of dependence

Airway Clearance, Ineffective
Related factors: Decreased energy/fatigue, Tracheobronchial obstruction, Tracheobronchial secretions

Aspiration: High Risk
Risk factor: Presence of tracheostomy or endotracheal tube

Body Image Disturbance
Related factor: Chronic illness

Breathing Pattern, Ineffective
Related factors: Decreased energy/fatigue, Anxiety

Caregiver Role Strain (Actual/High Risk)
Related factors/risk factors: Illness severity of the care receiver, Unpredicatable illness course or instability in the care receiver's health, Duration of caregiving required, Inadequate physical environment for providing care, Lack of respite and recreation for caregiver, Complexity/amount of caregiving tasks

Coping, Ineffective Individual
Related factor: Personal vulnerability in situational crisis (declining health)

Dysfunctional Ventilatory Weaning Response (DVWR)

Related factors: Ineffective airway clearance, Inadequate nutrition, Patient perceived inefficacy about the ability to wean, Decreased motivation, Decreased self-esteem, Anxiety, Inappropriate pacing of diminished ventilator support, Adverse environment, History of ventilatory dependence > 1 week, History of multiple unsuccessful weaning attempts.

Family Processes, Altered

Related factors: Change in family roles, Change in family structure, Hospitalization/change in environment, Illness/disability of family member

Fear

Related factors: Environmental stressors/hospitalization, Real or imagined threat to own well-being

Fluid Volume Deficit: High Risk

Risk factors: Inadequate fluid intake secondary to difficulty in breathing, Medications

Gas Exchange, Impaired

Related factor: Decreased functional lung tissue secondary to chronic lung disease

Health Maintenance, Altered

Related factors: Health beliefs, Lack of social supports

Infection: High Risk

Risk factors: Malnutrition, Environmental exposure to ___ (specify)

Knowledge Deficit (specify)

Related factors: Information misinterpretation, Limited exposure to information (specify)

Nutrition, Altered; Less Than Body Requirements

Related factors: Loss of appetite, Nausea/vomiting

Powerlessness

Related factors: Treatment regimen, Chronic illness

Role Performance, Altered

Related factor: Chronic illness

Self-Care Deficit: Bathing/Hygiene, Dressing/Grooming, Feeding, Toileting (specify)

Related factors: Decreased strength and endurance, Intolerance to activity

Self-Esteem Disturbance

Related factor: Chronic illness

Sleep Pattern Disturbance

Related factors: Anxiety, Medically induced regimen

Social Interaction, Impaired

Related factor: Self-concept disturbance

Therapeutic Regimen Management, Ineffective Individual

Related factors: Complexity of therapeutic regimen, Decisional conflict, Family patterns of health care, Knowledge deficits, Perceived seriousness, Powerlessness, Social support deficits

■ TERMINAL PATIENT

Activity Intolerance

Related factors: Chronic pain, Weakness/fatigue

Adjustment, Impaired

Related factors: Inadequate support systems, Incomplete grieving

Airway Clearance, Ineffective

Related factors: Decreased energy/fatigue, Pain, Tracheobronchial obstruction

Body Image Disturbance

Related factor: Treatment side-effects

Bowel Incontinence

Related factors: Loss of sphincter control, Decreased awareness of need to defecate

Breathing Pattern, Ineffective

Related factor: Chronic pain

**Caregiver Role Strain
(Actual/High Risk)**
Related factors/risk factors: Illness severity of the care receiver, Unpredicatable illness course or instability in the care receiver's health, Duration of caregiving required, Inadequate physical environment for providing care, Lack of respite and recreation for caregiver, Complexity/amount of caregiving tasks

Communication, Impaired: Verbal
Related factors: Inability to speak, Inability to speak clearly

Constipation
Related factors: Decreased activity, Decreased motility secondary to medications

**Coping, Ineffective Family:
Compromised**
Related factor: Family member's temporary preoccupation with own emotional conflicts and personal suffering

Coping, Ineffective Individual
Related factor: Personal vulnerability to situational crisis (terminal illness)

Denial, Ineffective
Related factor: Fear of consequences

Diarrhea
Related factor: Impaction

Family Processes, Altered
Related factors: Change in family roles, Hospitalization/change in environment, Illness/disability of family member

Fatigue
Related factors: Disease process, Overwhelming psychologic or emotional demands

Fear
Related factors: Powerlessness, Environmental stressors/hospitalization

Fluid Volume Deficit
Related factor: Inadequate fluid intake

Fluid Volume Deficit: High Risk
Risk factors: Excessive losses through normal routes, Loss of fluid through abnormal routes, Deviations affecting access to or intake or absorption of fluids

Gas Exchange, Impaired
Related factors: Decreased functional lung tissue, Decreased pulmonary blood supply

Grieving, Anticipatory
Related factor: Impending death of self

**Home Maintenance Management,
Impaired**
Related factors: Home environment obstacles, Inadequate support system, Insufficient family organization or planning, Insufficient finances, Lack of familiarity with community resources

Hopelessness
Related factors: Failing or deteriorating physical condition, Lack of social support

Infection: High Risk
Risk factors: Immunosuppression, Environmental exposure to ___ (specify)

Mobility, Impaired Physical
Related factors: Pain/discomfort, Decreased strength and endurance

**Nutrition, Altered: Less Than Body
Requirements**
Related factors: Difficulty in swallowing, Loss of appetite, Nausea/vomiting

Oral Mucous Membrane, Altered
Related factors: Chemotherapy, Inadequate oral hygiene, Radiation to head and neck

Pain, Chronic
Related factors: Specific to patient

Powerlessness
Related factor: Terminal illness

Role Performance, Altered
Related factors: Chronic pain, Treatment side-effects

Self-Care Deficit: Bathing/Hygiene, Dressing/Grooming, Feeding, Toileting (specify)
Related factors: Pain/discomfort, Intolerance to activity, Decreased strength and endurance

Self-Esteem Disturbance
Related factor: Treatment side-effects

Sensory/Perceptual Alterations: Visual, Auditory, Kinesthetic, Gustatory, Tactile, Olfactory (specify)
Related factors: Altered sensory reception, transmission, and/or integration

Skin Integrity, Impaired
Related factors: Physical immobilization, Incontinence stool/urine, Radiation therapy

Skin Integrity, Impaired: High Risk
Risk factors: Physical immobilization, Incontinence of stool/urine, Radiation therapy

Sleep Pattern Disturbance
Related factors: Sleep deprivation, Pain/discomfort

Social Isolation
Related factors: Medical condition, Alteration in physical appearance

Spiritual Distress
Related factors: Challenged belief and value system, Separation from religious/cultural ties, Test of spiritual beliefs

Urinary Incontinence, Functional
Related factors: Disorientation, Mobility deficit

Urinary Incontinence, Total
Related factor: Neurologic dysfunction

■ UROLOGIC DISORDERS

Includes but is not limited to cystitis, glomerulonephritis, pyelonephritis, urolithiasis.

Anxiety
Related factor: Threat to or change in health status

Fear
Related factor: Real or imagined threat to own well-being

Knowledge Deficit (specify)
Related factor: Limited exposure to information

Pain [Acute]
Related factor: Inflammation

Urinary Incontinence, Urge
Related factor: Bladder irritation

Urinary Retention
Related factors: Blockage, Strong sphincter, Inhibition of reflex arc, High urethral pressure caused by weak detrusor

■ VASCULAR DISEASE

Includes but is not limited to deep vein thrombosis, hypertension, stasis ulcers, varicosities, peripheral vascular disease, thrombophlebitis.

Activity Intolerance
Related factors: Weakness/fatigue, Acute pain

Anxiety
Related factors: Threat to or change in role functioning, Threat to or change in health status

Body Image Disturbance
Related factor: Chronic illness

Disuse Syndrome: High Risk
Risk factor: Prescribed immobilization

Fear
Related factor: Real or imagined threat to own well-being

Fluid Volume Deficit: High Risk
Risk factor: Medication

Injury: High Risk
Risk factors: Sensory dysfunction, Altered mobility

Mobility, Impaired Physical
Related factor: Pain/discomfort

Pain [Acute]
Related factor: Disease process

Role Performance, Altered
Related factor: Chronic pain

Self-Care Deficit: Bathing/Hygiene, Dressing/Grooming, Feeding, Toileting (specify)
Related factors: Pain/discomfort, Intolerance to activity

Self-Esteem Disturbance
Related factor: Chronic illness

Skin Integrity, Impaired
Related factors: Draining wound, Altered circulation, Physical immobilization

Skin Integrity, Impaired: High Risk
Risk factors: Draining wound, Altered circulation, Physical immobilization

Tissue Perfusion, Altered: Peripheral
Related factor: Impaired venous circulation

Surgical Conditions

Abdominal surgery
Breast surgery
Chest surgery
Craniotomy
Ear surgery
Eye surgery
Musculoskeletal surgery

Neck surgery
Rectal surgery
Skin graft
Spinal surgery
Urologic surgery
Vascular surgery

■ ABDOMINAL SURGERY

Includes but is not limited to appendectomy, cholecystectomy, colectomy, colon resection, colostomy, gastrectomy, gastric resection, gastroenterostomy, abdominal hysterectomy with or without salpingo-oophrectomy, ileostomy, laparotomy, lysis of adhesions, Marshall-Marchetti-Krantz operation, ovarian cystectomy, salpingotomy, small bowel resection, splenectomy, vagotomy, hiatal hernia repair.

Activity Intolerance
Related factors: Acute pain, Weakness/fatigue

Activity Intolerance: High Risk
Risk factors: Limited mobility, Pain, Fatigue

Aspiration: High Risk
Risk factors: Depressed cough and gag reflexes, Presence of endotracheal tube, Incomplete lower esophageal sphincter, Gastrointestinal tubes, Tube feedings, Increased intragastric pressure, Increased gastric residual, Decreased gastrointestinal motility, Delayed gastric emptying, Hindered elevation of upper body

Body Image Disturbance
Related factors: Surgery, Situational crisis, Treatment side-effects, Cultural or spiritual factors

Bowel Incontinence
Related factors: Loss of sphincter control

Breathing Pattern, Ineffective
Related factor: Pain

Caregiver Role Strain
Related factors: Illness severity of care receiver, Discharge of family member with significant home care needs, Past history of poor relationship between caregiver and care receiver

Constipation, Colonic
Related factors: Decreased activity, Decreased fluid intake, Lack of adequate fiber, Immobility, Lack of privacy, Change in daily routine

Diarrhea
Related factors: Dietary changes, Increased intestinal motility, Medication, Stress

Fear
Related factors: Environmental stressors/hospitalization, Powerlessness, Real or imagined threat to own well-being

Fluid Volume Deficit
Related factors: Abnormal blood loss, Abnormal fluid loss, Failure of regulatory mechanisms

Fluid Volume Deficit: High Rrisk
Risk factors: Excessive losses through normal routes, Loss of fluid through abnormal routes, Deviations affecting access to or intake or absorption of fluids

Gas Exchange, Impaired
Related factors: Decreased functional lung tissue secondary to atelectasis, Ventilation-perfusion imbalance

Grieving, Anticipatory
Related factor: Potential loss of body part or function

Grieving, Dysfunctional
Related factors: Actual loss, Terminal illness

Infection: High Risk
Risk factors: Stasis of body fluids, Altered peristalsis, Suppressed inflammatory response, Invasive procedures

Knowledge Deficit (specify)
Related factors: Limited practice of skill, Unreadiness to learn

Nutrition, Altered: Less Than Body Requirements
Related factors: Loss of appetite, Nausea/vomiting

Protection, Altered
Related factors: Deficient immunity secondary to ___, Impaired healing secondary to ___, Altered clotting secondary to ___

Role Performance, Altered
Related factors: Surgery, Situational crisis (specify), Treatment side-effects

Sexual Dysfunction
Related factors: Pain, Health-related transitions, Body image disturbance, Surgery, Altered body function or structure

Skin Integrity, Impaired: High Risk
Risk factors: Mechanical factors, Physical immobilization, Excretions/secretions, Alterations in nutritional state, Altered sensation, Skeletal prominence

Therapeutic Regimen Management, Ineffective Individual
Related factors: Complexity of therapeutic regimen, Economic difficulties, Knowledge deficits

Tissue Perfusion, Altered: Gastrointestinal
Related factors: Interruption of arterial flow, Exchange problems, Hypervolemia, Hypovolemia

■ BREAST SURGERY

Includes but is not limited to augmentation, mastectomy, reconstruction, lumpectomy, biopsy.

Activity Intolerance
Related factors: Acute pain, Anxiety

Anxiety
Related factors: Threat to self-concept, Threat to or change in health status, Threat to or change in interaction pattern, Situational/maturational crisis

Body Image Disturbance
Related factors: Surgery, Treatment side-effects, Cultural or spiritual factors

Caregiver Role Strain: High Risk
Risk factor: Caregiver is spouse

Family Processes, Altered
Related factors: Complex therapies, Hospitalization/change in environment

Fear
Related factors: Disease process/prognosis, Powerlessness, Real or imagined threat to own well-being

Grieving, Anticipatory
Related factor: Potential loss of body part or function

Pain [Acute]
Related factors: Surgical procedure, Paresthesia

Peripheral Neurovascular Dysfunction: High Risk
Risk factor: Vascular obstruction

Powerlessness
Related factor: Treatment regimen

Self-Care Deficit: Dressing/Grooming
Related factors: Pain/discomfort, Neuromuscular impairment

Sexual Dysfunction
Related factors: Surgery, Pain, Health-related transitions, Altered body function or structure, Illness/medical treatment, Body image disturbance, Self-esteem disturbance

■ CHEST SURGERY

Includes but is not limited to biopsy, cardiopulmonary bypass, coronary artery bypass, lobectomy, thoracotomy.

Activity Intolerance
Related factors: Imbalance between oxygen supply and demand, Acute pain, Weakness/fatigue

Activity Intolerance: High Risk
Risk factors: Limited mobility, Pain, Fatigue

Adjustment, Impaired
Related factor: Necessity for major lifestyle/behavior changes

Airway Clearance, Ineffective
Related factors: Decreased energy/fatigue, Tracheobronchial secretions

Aspiration: High Risk
Risk factor: Presence of endotracheal tube

Breathing Pattern, Ineffective
Related factors: Decreased energy/fatigue, Acute pain

Cardiac Output, Decreased
Related factors: Dysfunctional electrical conduction, Ventricular ischemia, Ventricular damage

Caregiver Role Strain
Related factors: Discharge of family member with significant home care needs, Caregivers competing role commitments

Communication, Impaired: Verbal
Related factor: Intubation

Coping, Ineffective Individual
Related factor: Personal vulnerability in situational crisis (specify)

Dysfunctional Ventilatory Weaning Response (DVWR)
Related factors: Uncontrolled pain/discomfort, Moderate/severe anxiety, Fear, History of ventilatory dependence <1 week

Fatigue
Related factors: Pain, Disease process

Fear
Related factors: Environmental stressors/hospitalization, Real or imagined threat to own well-being

Fluid Volume Deficit
Related factors: Abnormal fluid loss, Abnormal blood loss

Fluid Volume Deficit: High Risk
Risk factors: Excessive losses through normal routes, Loss of fluid through abnormal routes, Deviations affecting access to or intake or absorption of fluids

Gas Exchange, Impaired
Related factors: Decreased functional lung tissue secondary to pneumonia, thoracotomy, respiratory distress syndrome, Ventilation-perfusion imbalance

Noncompliance
Related factors: Denial of illness, Negative perception of treatment regimen

Pain [Acute]
Related factor: Surgical procedure

Powerlessness
Related factor: Treatment regimen

Protection, Altered
Related factor: Altered clotting secondary to ___

Role Performance, Altered
Related factors: Surgery, Treatment side-effects

Self-Care Deficit: Bathing/Hygiene, Dressing/Grooming (specify)
Related factors: Pain/discomfort, Intolerance to activity, Decreased strength and endurance

Skin Integrity, Impaired
Related factors: Altered circulation, Altered sensation, Mechanical factors

Sleep Pattern Disturbance
Related factors: Pain/discomfort, Unfamiliar surroundings, Medically induced regimen

■ CRANIOTOMY

Includes but is not limited to acoustic neuroma removal, cerebral aneurysm clipping, cerebral bleed, cerebral trauma.

Activity Intolerance
Related factor: Weakness/fatigue

Airway Clearance, Ineffective
Related factor: Tracheobronchial secretions

Body Image Disturbance
Related factors: Surgery, Treatment side-effects

Body Temperature, Altered: High Risk
Risk factors: Altered metabolic rate, Trauma, Sedation

Bowel Incontinence
Related factor: Decreased awareness of need to defecate

Breathing Pattern, Ineffective
Related factors: Depression of respiratory center secondary to ___, Neuromuscular paralysis/weakness

Caregiver Role Strain: High Risk
Risk factors: Illness severity of care receiver, Discharge of family member with significant home care needs, Unpredictable illness course, Psychologic or cognitive problems in care receiver

Communication, Impaired: Verbal
Related factors: Aphasia, Acute confusion, Intubation

Coping, Ineffective Individual
Related factor: Personal vulnerability in situational crisis (specify)

Disuse Syndrome: High Risk
Risk factors: Paralysis, Mechanical immobilization, Prescribed immobilization, Altered level of consciousness

Fear
Related factors: Environmental stressors/hospitalization, Powerlessness, Real or imagined threat to own well-being

Fluid Volume Deficit
Related factor: Failure of regulatory mechanisms (diabetes insipidus)

Fluid Volume Deficit: High Risk
Risk factors: Excessive losses through normal routes, Loss of fluid through abnormal routes, Deviations affecting access to or intake or absorption of fluids

Fluid Volume Excess
Related factor: Decreased urine output secondary to renal dysfunction

Injury: High Risk
Risk factor: Sensory dysfunction

Mobility, Impaired Physical
Related factors: Neuromuscular impairment, Perceptual/cognitive impairment, Depression/severe anxiety

Pain [Acute]
Related factors: Surgical procedure, Paresthesia

Peripheral Neurovascular Dysfunction: High Risk
Related factors: Trauma, Vascular obstruction

Protection, Altered
Related factors: Neurosensory alterations secondary to ___, Altered clotting secondary to ___ (specify)

Role Performance, Altered
Related factors: Surgery, Psychologic impairment, Treatment side-effects, Assumption of new role

Self-Care Deficit: Bathing/Hygiene, Dressing/Grooming, Feeding, Toileting (specify)
Related factors: Intolerance to activity, Neuromuscular impairment

Sensory/Perceptual Alterations: Visual, Auditory, Kinesthetic, Gustatory, Tactile, Olfactory (specify)
Related factors: Altered sensory reception, transmission, and/or integration, Sensory deficit, Sensory overload

Swallowing, Impaired
Related factors: Altered sensory reception, transmission, and/or integration, Neuromuscular impairment

Tissue Perfusion, Altered: Cerebral
Related factor: Interruption of arterial flow

Urinary Incontinence, Functional
Related factors: Cognitive impairment, Disorientation, Mobility deficits

Urinary Incontinence, Total

Related factors: Neuropathy preventing transmissions of reflex indicating bladder fullness, Neurologic dysfunction causing triggering of micturition at unpredictable times, Independent contraction of detrusor reflex due to surgery

■ EAR SURGERY

Includes but is not limited to myringotomy, reconstruction, stapedectomy.

Body Image Disturbance
Related factor: Surgery

Fear
Related factor: Real or imagined threat to own well-being

Mobility, Impaired Physical
Related factor: Neuromuscular impairment

Self-Care Deficit: Bathing/Hygiene, Dressing/Grooming, Feeding, Toileting (specify)
Related factor: Intolerance to activity secondary to dizziness

Sensory/Perceptual Alterations: Auditory, Tactile
Related factors: Sensory deficit, Sensory overload

■ EYE SURGERY

Includes but is not limited to blepharoplasty, cataract removal, cryosurgery for retinal detachment, iridectomy, iridotomy, lens implant.

Body Image Disturbance
Related factor: Surgery

Fear
Related factor: Real or imagined threat to own well-being

Injury: High Risk
Risk factors: Sensory deficit, Unsafe ambulation secondary to limited vision

Mobility, Impaired Physical
Related factor: Medically prescribed treatment

Sensory/Perceptual Alteration: Visual
Related factor: Sensory deficit

Tissue Integrity, Impaired
Related factor: Irritants

■ MUSCULOSKELETAL SURGERY

Includes but is not limited to amputation, arthrotomy, bunionectomy, casts, hip pinning, hip prosthesis, open reduction/internal fixation of fracture, shoulder repair, total ankle replacement, total hip replacement, total knee replacement, traction.

Activity Intolerance
Related factors: Acute pain, Weakness/fatigue

Adjustment, Impaired
Related factor: Necessity for major lifestyle/behavior change

Anxiety
Related factors: Threat to self-concept, Threat to or change in health status, Threat to or change in role functioning

Body Image Disturbance
Related factors: Surgery, Treatment side-effects

Caregiver Role Strain: High Risk
Risk factors: Illness severity of care receiver, Presence of situational stressors, Duration of caregiving required

Constipation
Related factors: Decreased activity, Dietary changes, Medication

Disuse Syndrome: High Risk
Risk factor: Prescribed immobilization

Diversional Activity Deficit
Related factor: Prolonged bed rest

Fatigue
Related factor: Increased energy requirement to perform activities of daily living

Fluid Volume Deficit: High Risk
Risk factors: Excessive losses through normal routes, Loss of fluid through abnormal routes, Deviations affecting access to or intake or absorption of fluids

Injury: High Risk
Risk factor: Altered mobility

Mobility, Impaired Physical
Related factors: Pain/discomfort, Medically prescribed limitations, Decreased strength and endurance

Nutrition, Altered: More Than Body Requirements
Related factors: Lack of physical exercise, Decreased metabolic requirements

Pain [Acute]
Related factors: Muscle cramps, Paresthesia

Peripheral Neurovascular Dysfunction: High Risk
Risk factors: Fractures, Mechanical compression, Orthopedic surgery, Trauma, Immobilization

Relocation Stress Syndrome
Related factors: Feeling of powerlessness, Decreased physical health status

Role Performance, Altered
Related factors: Surgery, Situational crisis, Chronic pain

Self-Care Deficit: Bathing/Hygiene, Dressing/Grooming, Feeding, Toileting (specify)
Related factors: Pain/discomfort, Intolerance to activity, Decreased strength and endurance

Skin Integrity, Impaired: High Risk
Risk factors: Mechanical factors, Physical immobilization, Altered circulation, Altered sensation

Sleep Pattern Disturbance
Related factors: Pain/discomfort, Unfamiliar surroundings, Medically induced regimen

Tissue Perfusion, Altered: Peripheral
Related factors: Interruption of arterial flow, Interruption of venous flow

■ NECK SURGERY

Includes but is not limited to carotid endarterectomy, laryngectomy, parathyroidectomy, radical neck dissection, thyroidectomy, tonsillectomy, tracheostomy.

Activity Intolerance
Related factors: Imbalance between oxygen supply and demand, Anxiety, Acute pain, Weakness/fatigue

Activity Intolerance: High Risk
Risk factors: Limited mobility, Fatigue

Adjustment, Impaired
Related factors: Assault to self-esteem, Necessity for major life-style/behavior change

Airway Clearance, Ineffective
Related factors: Decreased energy/fatigue, Edema, Pain, Tracheobronchial obstruction, Tracheobronchial secretions

Aspiration: High Risk
Risk factors: Depressed cough or gag reflex, Presence of tracheostomy or endotracheal tube, Impaired swallowing, Hindered elevation of upper body

Body Image Disturbance
Related factors: Surgery, Depression, Treatment side-effects

Breathing Pattern, Ineffective
Related factors: Anxiety, Decreased energy/fatigue

Caregiver Role Strain: High Risk
Risk factors: Illness severity of care receiver, Duration of caregiving required, Inadequate physical environment for providing care, Complexity/amount of caregiving tasks

Communication, Impaired: Verbal
Related factors: Acute confusion,
Inability to speak, Inability to speak
clearly, Tracheostomy

Coping, Ineffective Individual
Related factor: Personal vulnerability in
situational crisis (specify)

**Dysfunctional Ventilatory Weaning
Response (DVWR)**
Related factors: Ineffective airway
clearance, Decreased motivation,
Moderate/severe anxiety, Fear, Uncontrolled episodic energy demands or
problems

Family Processes, Altered
Related factors: Change in family roles,
Illness/disability of family member

Fear
Related factors: Real or imagined threat
to own well-being, Powerlessness

Fluid Volume Deficit: High Risk
Risk factors: Loss of fluid through
abnormal routes, Hypermetabolic state

Fluid Volume Excess
Related factor: Insufficient protein
secondary to decreased intake

Grieving, Dysfunctional
Related factor: Actual loss

Infection: High Risk
Risk factors: Tissue destruction and
increased environmental exposure,
Trauma

Injury: High Risk
Risk factors: Sensory dysfunction,
Integrative dysfunction, Altered mobility

Knowledge Deficit (specify)
Related factors: Lack of motivation,
Limited practice of skill (specify),
Unreadiness to learn

**Nutrition, Altered: Less Than Body
Requirements**
Related factors: Difficulty in swallowing, High metabolic states, Loss of
appetite, Nausea/vomiting

Oral Mucous Membrane, Altered
Related factors: Inadequate oral
hygiene, Tubes, Surgery in oral cavity,
Infection, Radiation therapy to head
and neck

Pain [Acute]
Related factor: Surgical procedure

Role Performance, Altered
Related factors: Surgery, Treatment
side-effects

Skin Integrity, Impaired
Related factors: Mechanical factors,
Radiation, Altered nutritional state

**Spontaneous Ventilation, Inability to
Sustain**
Related factor: Respiratory muscle
fatigue

Swallowing, Impaired
Related factors: Irritated oropharyngeal
cavity, Mechanical obstruction

Tissue Integrity, Impaired
Related factors: Nutritional deficit,
Irritants, Mechanical factors, Radiation

■ RECTAL SURGERY

Includes but is not limited to
fissurectomy, hemorrhoidectomy,
pilonidal cystectomy, polypectomy.

Activity Intolerance
Related factor: Acute pain

Constipation
Related factors: Dietary changes,
Medication, Painful defecation

Pain [Acute]
Related factor: Surgical procedure

Sexual Dysfunction
Related factors: Surgery, Pain, Disease,
Health-related transitions, Altered body
function, Trauma

Tissue Integrity, Impaired
Related factors: Altered circulation,
Irritants, Mechanical factors

Urinary Rretention
Related factors: Inhibition of reflex arc, Blockage

■ SKIN GRAFT

Includes but is not limited to excision of lesion with flap, excision of lesion with full thickness graft, excision of lesion with split thickness graft, excision of lesion with synthetic graft.

Activity Intolerance
Related factors: Anxiety, Weakness/fatigue, Decreased activity

Body Image Disturbance
Related factors: Surgery, Treatment side-effects

Constipation
Related factor: Decreased activity

Diversional Activity Deficit
Related factor: Prolonged bed rest

Fear
Related factors: Powerlessness, Real or imagined threat to own well-being

Mobility, Impaired Physical
Related factors: Pain/discomfort, Medically prescribed limitations

Pain [Acute]
Related factors: Surgical procedure, Pruritus, Paresthesia

Peripheral Neurovascular Dysfunction: High Risk
Risk factors: Immobilization, Burns

■ SPINAL SURGERY

Includes but is not limited to Harrington rod implant, laminectomy, Luque rod implant, spinal fusion.

Activity Intolerance
Related factors: Anxiety, Acute pain, Weakness/fatigue, Sedentary life-style

Caregiver Role Strain: High Risk
Risk factors: Premature birth/congenital defect, Developmental delay or retardation of the care receiver/caregiver, Duration of caregiving required

Constipation, Colonic
Related factors: Decreased activity, Medication, Painful defecation, Change in daily routine

Disuse Syndrome: High Risk
Risk factor: Prescribed immobilization

Dysreflexia
Related factors: Urinary retention, Constipation

Fear
Related factor: Real or imagined threat to own well-being

Fluid Volume Deficit: High Risk
Risk factors: Excessive losses through normal routes, Loss of fluid through abnormal routes, Deviations affecting access to or intake or absorption of fluids

Injury: High Risk
Risk factors: Sensory dysfunction, Altered mobility

Mobility, Impaired Physical
Related factors: Pain/discomfort, Medically prescribed limitations, Neuromuscular impairment

Nutrition, Altered: More Than Body Requirements
Related factors: Increased appetite, Sedentary life-style, Decreased activity

Pain [Acute]
Related factors: Bed rest, Muscle cramps, Paresthesia, Surgical procedure

Pain, Chronic
Related factors: Neurologic injury, Altered body function

Peripheral Neurovascular Dysfunction: High Risk
Risk factors: Fractures, Mechanical compression, Trauma, Immobilization

Role Performance, Altered
Related factors: Surgery, Chronic pain, Chronic illness

■ UROLOGIC SURGERY

Includes but is not limited to cystocele repair, rectocele repair, removal of bladder tumor, cystoscopy, nephrostomy, penile implant, percutaneous nephrostomy, retroperitoneal lymphadenotomy, transurethral resection of the prostate, ureterolithotomy, urostomy, vasectomy.

Activity Intolerance
Related factors: Anxiety, Acute pain, Weakness/fatigue

Anxiety
Related factors: Threat to self-concept, Threat to or change in health status, Threat to or change in role functioning, Threat to or change in interaction pattern

Body Image Disturbance
Related factors: Surgery, Depression, Treatment side-effects

Caregiver Role Strain: High Risk
Risk factors: Discharge of family member with significant home care needs, Caregiver is female, Caregiver is spouse, Duration of caregiving required

Constipation
Related factor: Painful defecation

Fear
Related factor: Real or imagined threat to own well-being

Fluid Volume Deficit
Related factors: Abnormal fluid loss, Inadequate fluid intake

Fluid Volume Deficit: High Risk
Risk factor: Loss of fluid through abnormal route

Grieving, Anticipatory
Related factor: Potential loss of body parts or function

Grieving, Dysfunctional
Related factor: Perceived loss

Infection: High Risk
Risk factors: Stasis of body fluids, Change in pH secretions, Decreased hemoglobin, Suppressed inflammatory response, Tissue destruction and increased environmental exposure, Invasive procedures

Mobility, Impaired Physical
Related factors: Pain, Discomfort

Pain [Acute]
Related factors: Muscle cramps, Surgical procedure

Role Performance, Altered
Related factors: Surgery, Psychologic impairment

Sexual Dysfunction
Related factors: Surgery, Pain, Health-related transitions, Altered body function or structure, Body image disturbance

Urinary Incontinence, Stress
Related factors: Incompetent bladder outlet, Overdistention between voidings, Weak pelvic muscles and structural supports

Urinary Incontinence, Urge
Related factors: Decreased bladder capacity, Surgery, Irritation of bladder stretch receptors causing spasm, Overdistention of bladder

Urinary Retention
Related factors: Inhibition of reflex arc, Blockage

■ VASCULAR SURGERY

Includes but is not limited to aortic
aneurysm resection, aorto-iliac bypass
graft, embolectomy, femoro-iliac bypass
graft, portacaval shunt, sympathectomy,
vein ligation.

Activity Intolerance
Related factors: Anxiety, Acute pain,
Weakness/fatigue, Imbalance between
oxygen supply and demand

Adjustment, Impaired
Related factor: Necessity for major life-
style/behavior change

Cardiac Output, Decreased
Related factors: Dysfunctional electrical
conduction, Ventricular ischemia,
Ventricular damage

Caregiver Role Strain: High Risk
Risk factors: Illness severity of care
receiver, Unpredictable illness course or
instability in the care receiver's health,
Complexity/amount of caregiving tasks

Fear
Related factor: Real or imagined threat
to own well-being

Fluid Volume Deficit: High Risk
Risk factors: Loss of fluid through
abnormal routes, Medications

Fluid Volume Excess
Related factor: Decreased urine output
secondary to heart failure

Gas Exchange, Impaired
Related factor: Decreased functional
lung tissue, Decreased pulmonary blood
supply

Grieving, Anticipatory
Related factor: Potential loss of body
part or function

Grieving, Dysfunctional
Related factor: Perceived loss

Injury: High Risk
Risk factors: Tissue hypoxia, Abnormal
blood profile, Altered mobility

Pain [Acute]
Related factor: Surgical procedure

Peripheral Neurovascular Dysfunction: High Risk
Risk factors: Immobilization, Vascular
obstruction

Role Performance, Altered
Related factors: Surgery, Chronic illness,
Treatment side-effects, Assumption of
new role

Self-Esteem Disturbance
Related factors: Surgery, Depression

Tissue Perfusion, Altered: Renal, Cerebral, Cardiopulmonary, Gastrointestinal, Peripheral (specify type)
Related factors: Interruption of venous
flow, Exchange problems

Psychiatric Conditions

Assaultive patient
Borderline personality disorder
   patient
Chronically ill psychiatric
   patient
Eating disorder patient
Manic patient

Paranoid patient
Phobic patient
Psychotic patient
Severely depressed patient
Substance abuse patient
Suicidal patient
Withdrawn patient

■ ASSAULTIVE PATIENT

Associated psychiatric diagnoses include but are not limited to bipolar disorder, manic; schizophrenia, disorganized type; substance abuse disorders; organic mental disorders; drug-induced psychoses; personality disorders; panic disorders; post-traumatic stress disorder.

Coping, Defensive
Related factors: Psychologic impairment (specify), Situational crisis (specify)

Denial, Ineffective
Related factor: Specific to patient

Fear
Related factors: Real or imagined threat to own well-being, Powerlessness

Personal Identity Disturbance
Related factors: Situational crisis (specify), Psychologic impairment (specify)

Post-Trauma Response
Related factors: Abuse, Incest, Rape, Participation in combat

Role Performance, Altered
Related factors: Situational crises (specify), Psychologic impairment (specify)

Self-Esteem, Low: Chronic
Related factors: Psychologic impairment (specify), Repeatedly unmet expectations

Self-Esteem, Low: Situational
Related factor: Situational crisis (specify)

Sensory/Perceptual Alterations: Visual, Auditory, Kinesthetic, Gustatory, Tactile, Olfactory (specify)
Related factors: Alcohol/substance abuse (specify), Altered sensory reception, transmission, and/or integration, Sensory deficit (specify), Sensory overload

Social Interaction, Impaired
Related factors: Developmental disability, Communication barriers, Psychologic impairment (specify)

Thought Processes, Altered
Related factors: Mental disorder (specify), Organic mental disorder (specify), Personality disorder (specify), Substance abuse

Violence, High Risk: Self-Directed or Directed at Others
Risk factors: Manic excitement, Panic states, Rage reaction, History of violence, Drug/alcohol intoxication/withdrawal, Temporal lobe epilepsy, Paranoid ideation, Organic brain syndrome, Arrest/conviction pattern, Toxic reaction to medications, Command hallucinations

■ BORDERLINE PERSONALITY DISORDER PATIENT

Anxiety
Related factors: Threat to role functioning, Change in role functioning, Situational crises (specify), Maturational crisis (specify), Unmet needs, Threat to or change in environment, Threat to or change in interaction patterns

Coping, Ineffective Family: Disabling
Related factors: Conflicting coping styles, Highly ambivalent family relationships, Chronically unresolved feelings (specify)

Coping, Ineffective Individual
Related factors: Personal vulnerability in situational crisis (specify), Personal vulnerability in maturational crisis (specify)

Decisional Conflict
Related factors: Specific to patient

Parenting, Altered
Related factor: Psychologic impairment (borderline personality disorder)

Personal Identity Disturbance
Related factors: Situational crises, Psychologic impairment (borderline personality disorder)

Post-Trauma Response
Related factors: Abuse, Incest, Rape

Powerlessness
Related factor: Pattern of helplessness

Role Performance, Altered
Related factors: Situational crises,
Psychologic impairment (borderline
personality disorder)

Self-Esteem, Low Chronic
Related factors: Psychologic impairment
(borderline personality disorder),
Repeatedly unmet expectations

Self-Mutilation: High Risk
Risk factors: Inability to cope with
increased psychologic/physiologic
tension in a healthy manner, Feelings of
depression, rejection, self-hatred,
separation anxiety, guilt, and
depersonalization, Fluctuating emotions,
Drug/alcohol abuse, History of self-
injury, History of physical, emotional,
or sexual abuse

Sexuality Patterns, Altered
Related factors: Conflict with sexual
orientation, Sexual abuse, Impaired
relationship with significant person

Social Interaction, Impaired
Related factor: Psychologic impairment
(borderline personality disorder)

Thought Processes, Altered
Related factors: Psychologic impairment
(borderline personality disorder),
Substance abuse

**Violence, High Risk: Self-Directed or
Directed at Others**
Risk factors: Rage reaction, Suicidal
ideation, History of self-mutilation,
Substance abuse (specify)

■ CHRONICALLY ILL
PSYCHIATRIC PATIENT

Associated psychiatric diagnoses include but
are not limited to schizophrenia: disorganized
type, paranoid type, undifferentiated type;
affective disorders: bipolar disorder, major
depression (recurrent); eating disorders:
anorexia and bulimia; borderline personality
disorder; organic mental disorders; substance
abuse disorders.

**Caregiver Role Strain
(Actual/High Risk)**
Related factors/risk factors: Unpredictable illness course or instability in the
care receiver's health, Marginal
caregiver's coping patterns, Past history
of poor relationship between caregiver
and care receiver, Marginal family
adaptation or dysfunction prior to the
caregiving situation, Psychological
problems in care receiver, Care receiver
exhibits deviant, bizarre behavior,
Presence of abuse or violence, Duration
of caregiving required, Inexperience
with caregiving

Constipation, Colonic
Related factors: Medications, Decreased
activity, Chronic use of laxatives/enemas

Constipation, Perceived
Related factor: Impaired thought
processes

Coping, Ineffective Family: Disabling
Related factors: Arbitrary disregard for
patient's needs, Chronically unresolved
feelings (specify guilt, anxiety, hostility,
despair, etc.), Conflicting coping styles,
Highly ambivalent family relationships

Denial, Ineffective
Related factors: Specific to patient

Diversional Activity Deficit
Related factors: Deficit in social skills,
Disturbance in motivation, Impaired
perception of reality

Fluid Volume Excess
Related factor: Increased fluid intake
secondary to compulsive water drinking,
medications

Health Maintenance, Altered
Related factors: Lack of ability to make deliberate and thoughtful judgments, Lack of material resources, Lack of social supports

Home Maintenance Management, Impaired
Related factors: Psychologic impairment (specify), Insufficient family organization or planning, Insufficient finances, Inadequate support system, Lack of knowledge

Injury: High risk
Risk factors: Psychologic: Affective factors, Orientation; Chemical: Drugs (alcohol, caffeine, nicotine); Physical: Exploitation by others

Knowledge Deficit (specify)
Related factors: Information misinterpretation, Lack of motivation, Unreadiness to learn, Limited practice of skill (specify)

Noncompliance
Related factors: Denial of illness, Negative consequence of treatment regimen, Negative perception of treatment regimen, Perceived benefits of continued illness

Nutrition, Altered: Less Than Body Requirements
Related factors: Chemical dependence (specify), Psychologic impairment (specify), Economic factors

Nutrition, Altered: More Than Body Requirements
Related factors: Decreased metabolic requirements secondary to medication, Lack of physical exercise, Eating disorder (bulimia)

Parenting, Altered
Related factors: Psychologic impairment (specify), Lack of cognitive functioning, Substance abuse (specify), Unmet maturational needs of parent, Physical/emotional abuse of parent

Powerlessness
Related factors: Chronic illness, Pattern of helplessness

Self-Care Deficit: Bathing/Hygiene, Dressing/Grooming, Feeding, Toileting (specify)
Related factors: Psychologic impairment (specify), Depression, Severe anxiety

Self-Esteem, Low: Chronic
Related factors: Repeatedly unmet expectations, Psychologic impairment (specify)

Sensory/Perceptual Alterations: Visual, Auditory, Kinesthetic, Gustatory, Tactile, Olfactory (specify)
Related factors: Alcohol/substance abuse (specify), Electrolyte imbalance secondary to anorexia

Sexuality Patterns, Altered
Related factors: Lack of significant other, Conflicts with sexual orientation, Disturbance in self-esteem, Body image disturbance, Impaired relationship with significant other

Sleep Pattern Disturbance
Related factors: Anxiety, Inactivity, Psychologic impairment (specify)

Social Interaction, Impaired
Related factors: Self-concept disturbance, Psychologic impairment (specify), Chemical dependency (specify), Absence of significant other/peer

Social Isolation
Related factor: Psychologic impairment (specify)

Therapeutic Regimen Management, Ineffective Individual
Related factors: Complexity of health care system, Complexity of therapeutic regimen, Decisional Conflict, Economic difficulties, Family conflict, Mistrust of regimen and/or health care personnel, Perceived seriousness, Perceived benefits, Powerlessness, Social support deficits

Thought Processes, Altered
Related factors: Mental disorder (specify), Organic mental disorder (specify), Personality disorder (specify), Substance abuse

Violence, High Risk: Self-Directed or Directed at Others

Risk factors: History of violence, Panic states, Substance abuse (specify), History of suicide attempts, Arrest/conviction pattern

■ **EATING DISORDER PATIENT**

Associated psychiatric diagnoses are limited to anorexia nervosa and bulimia.

Activity Intolerance

Related factor: Weakness/fatigue

Anxiety

Related factors: Threat to self concept, Threat to or change in role functioning, Threat to or change in environment, Situational/maturational crises, Unmet needs

Body Image Disturbance

Related factor: Eating disorder

Body Temperature, Altered: High Risk

Risk factors: Extremes of weight, Inactivity, Vigorous activity, Altered metabolic rate

Constipation

Related factor: Dietary changes

Constipation, Colonic

Related factors: Less than adequate amounts of fiber and bulk-forming foods in diet, Chronic use of medication and enemas

Constipation, Perceived

Related factor: Impaired thought processes

Coping, Ineffective Family: Disabling

Related factors: Arbitrary disregard for patient's needs, Chronically unresolved feelings (specify guilt, anxiety, hostility, despair, and so on), Conflicting coping styles, Highly ambivalent family relationships

Coping, Ineffective Individual

Related factor: Personal vulnerability in a maturational or situational crisis (specify)

Denial, Ineffective

Related factors: Specific to patient

Diarrhea

Related factor: Dietary changes

Fatigue

Related factor: Altered body chemistry

Fear

Related factors: Powerlessness, Real or imagined threat to well-being

Fluid Volume Deficit: High Risk

Risk factor: Extremes of weight

Fluid Volume Excess

Related factor: Insufficient protein secondary to decreased intake

Infection: High Risk

Risk factors: Altered peristalsis, Malnutrition

Knowledge Deficit (specify)

Related factor: Limited exposure to information (i.e., balanced diet, meal planning)

Noncompliance

Related factors: Denial of illness, Negative perception of treatment regimen, Perceived benefits of continued illness

Nutrition, Altered: Less Than Body Requirements

Related factor: Psychologic impairment (bulimia, anorexia)

Nutrition, Altered: More Than Body Requirements

Related factor: Psychologic impairment (bulimia)

Oral Mucous Membrane, Altered

Related factor: Malnutrition

Post-Trauma Response

Related factors: Abuse, Incest

Powerlessness

Related factor: Chronic illness

Role Performance, Altered

Related factor: Psychologic impairment (eating disorder)

Self-Esteem, Low: Chronic
Related factors: Psychologic impairment (specify), Repeatedly unmet expectations

Sexuality Patterns, Altered
Related factors: Ineffective or absent role models, Body image disturbance, Impaired relationship with significant other, Disturbance in self-esteem

Social Interaction, Impaired
Related factor: Psychologic impairment (anorexia, bulimia)

Therapeutic Regimen Management, Ineffective Individual
Related factors: Decisional Conflict, Family conflict, Mistrust of regimen and/or health care personnel, Perceived seriousness, Perceived benefits, Powerlessness

Thought Processes, Altered
Related factor: Mental disorder (anorexia, bulimia)

■ MANIC PATIENT

Associated psychiatric diagnoses include but are not limited to bipolar disorders (manic, mixed), manic episode, schizophrenia (undifferentiated type, catatonic type), schizoaffective disorder, substance abuse disorders.

Anxiety
Related factors: Change in role functioning, Change in environment, Change in interaction patterns, Unmet needs

Coping, Defensive
Related factor: Psychologic impairment (specify)

Coping, Ineffective Individual
Related factor: Personal vulnerability in a situational crisis (specify)

Denial, Ineffective
Related factors: Specific to patient

Diarrhea
Related factor: Medications (lithium)

Family Processes, Altered
Related factor: Illness/disability of family member

Fluid Volume Deficit
Related factor: Inadequate fluid intake

Fluid Volume Excess
Related factor: Increased fluid intake secondary to lithium therapy

Health Maintenance, Altered
Related factors: Significant alteration in communication skills, Lack of ability to make deliberate and thoughtful judgments

Home Maintenance Management, Impaired
Related factor: Psychologic impairment (specify)

Injury: High Risk
Risk factors: Psychologic: Affective factors, Orientation; Chemical: Drugs (alcohol, caffeine, nicotine); Physical: Cognitive, affective, and psychomotor factors

Noncompliance
Related factors: Denial of illness, Negative perception of treatment regimen

Nutrition, Altered: Less Than Body Requirements
Related factor: Psychologic impairment (specify)

Parenting, Altered
Related factor: Psychologic impairment (specify)

Personal Identity Disturbance
Related factor: Psychologic impairment (specify)

Role Performance, Altered
Related factor: Psychologic impairment (specify)

Self-Care Deficit: Bathing/Hygiene, Dressing/Grooming, Feeding, Toileting (specify)
Related factor: Psychologic impairment (specify)

Sexuality Patterns, Altered
Related factor: Psychologic impairment
(specify)

Sleep Pattern Disturbance
Related factors: Psychologic impairment
(specify), Sleep deprivation

Social Interaction, Impaired
Related factor: Psychologic impairment
(specify)

Thought Processes, Altered
Related factor: Mental disorder (specify)

**Violence, High Risk: Self-Directed or
Directed at Others**
Risk factors: Manic excitement, Rage
reaction, History of violence, Command
hallucinations, Toxic reaction to
medications

■ PARANOID PATIENT

Associated psychiatric diagnoses include but
are not limited to schizophrenia: undifferentiated type, paranoid type; affective disorders:
major depression (single episode, recurrent),
bipolar disorders (mixed, manic, depressed),
schizoaffective disorder; paranoid disorders;
substance abuse disorders; organic mental
disorders; personality disorders.

Anxiety
Related factors: Threat to or change in
role functioning, Change in environment, Threat to or change in interaction
pattern

Coping, Defensive
Related factor: Psychologic impairment
(specify)

Coping, Ineffective Individual
Related factor: Personal vulnerability in
situational crisis

Family Processes, Altered
Related factor: Illness/disability of
family member

Fear
Related factor: Imagined threat to own
well-being

Health Maintenance, Altered
Related factors: Significant alteration in
communication skills, Lack of ability
to make deliberate and thoughtful
judgments

**Home Maintenance Management,
Impaired**
Related factor: Psychologic impairment
(specify)

Noncompliance
Related factors: Denial of illness,
Negative perception of treatment
regimen

**Nutrition, Altered: Less Than Body
Requirements**
Related factor: Psychologic impairment
(specify)

Parenting, Altered
Related factor: Psychologic impairment
(specify)

Personal Identity Disturbance
Related factor: Psychologic impairment
(specify)

Post-Trauma Response
Related factors: Abuse, Incest, Rape

Powerlessness
Related factors: Health care environment, Treatment regimen

Role Performance, Altered
Related factor: Psychologic impairment
(specify)

**Self-Care Deficit: Bathing/Hygiene,
Dressing/Grooming, Feeding,
Toileting (specify)**
Related factor: Psychologic impairment
(specify)

Self-Esteem Disturbance
Related factor: Psychologic impairment
(specify)

Sexuality Patterns, Altered
Related factors: Impaired relationship
with significant other, Conflicts with
sexual orientation

Sleep Pattern Disturbance
Related factor: Psychologic impairment

Social Interaction, Impaired
Related factor: Psychologic impairment
(specify)

Thought Processes, Altered
Related factors: Mental disorder
(specify), Organic mental disorder
(specify), Personality disorder (specify)

**Violence, High Risk: Self-Directed or
Directed at Others**
Risk factors: Panic states, Drug/alcohol
intoxication/withdrawal, Paranoid
ideation, Organic brain syndrome,
Command hallucinations

■ PHOBIC PATIENT

Associated psychiatric diagnoses include but
are not limited to agoraphobia, simple
phobia, social phobia.

Anxiety
Related factors: Threat to or change in
role functioning, Threat to or change in
environment, Threat to self-concept,
Threat to or change in interaction
pattern, Unmet needs

Coping, Ineffective Individual
Related factors: Personal vulnerability in
situational crisis (specify), Personal
vulnerability in maturational crisis
(specify)

Denial, Ineffective
Related factors: Specific to patient

Diversional Activity Deficit
Related factor: Impaired perception of
reality

Family Processes, Altered
Related factor: Illness of family member

Fear
Related factor: Real or imagined threat
to own well-being

Post-Trauma Response
Related factors: Abuse, Assault, Accidents, Disaster, Incest, Rape

Powerlessness
Related factor: Phobic disorder

Rape-Trauma Syndrome
Related factor: Biopsychosocial response
to event

Role Performance, Altered
Related factor: Psychologic impairment
(phobic disorder)

Social Interaction, Impaired
Related factor: Psychologic impairment
(phobic disorder)

Social Isolation
Related factor: Psychologic impairment
(phobic disorder)

Thought Processes, Altered
Related factor: Mental disorder (phobic
disorder)

■ PSYCHOTIC PATIENT

Associated psychiatric diagnoses include but
are not limited to schizophrenia: disorganized
type, catatonic type, paranoid type, undifferentiated type; schizophreniform disorder;
affective disorders: manic episode, major
depressive episode, bipolar disorders (mixed,
manic, depressed); organic mental disorders;
substance abuse disorders.

Communication, Impaired: Verbal
Related factor: Psychologic impairment
(specify)

Coping, Defensive
Related factor: Psychologic impairment
(specify)

Denial, Ineffective
Related factors: Specific to patient

Diversional Activity Deficit
Related factors: Disturbance in motivation, Impaired perception of reality

Family Processes, Altered
Related factors: Hospitalization/change
in environment, Illness/disability of
family member

Health Maintenance, Altered
Related factors: Lack of ability to make deliberate and thoughtful judgments

Home Maintenance Management, Impaired
Related factor: Psychologic impairment (specify)

Injury: High Risk
Risk factors: Psychologic: Affective factors, Orientation; Chemical: Drugs (alcohol, caffeine, nicotine); Physical: Cognitive, affective, and psychomotor factors

Noncompliance
Related factors: Denial of illness, Negative perception of treatment regimen

Parenting, Altered
Related factor: Psychologic impairment (specify)

Personal Identity Disturbance
Related factor: Psychologic impairment (specify)

Role Performance, Altered
Related factor: Psychologic impairment (specify)

Self-Care Deficit: Bathing/Hygiene, Dressing/Grooming, Feeding, Toileting (specify)
Related factor: Psychologic impairment (specify)

Self-Esteem Disturbance
Related factor: Psychologic impairment (specify)

Self-Mutilation: High Risk
Risk factors: Fluctuating emotions, Command hallucinations, Clients in psychotic state—frequently males in young adulthood

Sleep Pattern Disturbance
Related factor: Psychologic impairment (specify)

Social Interaction
Related factor: Psychologic impairment (specify)

Thought Processes, Altered
Related factors: Mental disorder (specify), Organic mental disorder (specify)

Violence, High Risk: Self-Directed or Directed at Others
Risk factors: Paranoid ideation, Suicide ideation, History of violence, Substance abuse (specify)

■ **SEVERELY DEPRESSED PATIENT**

Associated psychiatric diagnoses include but are not limited to bipolar disorder, depressed; major depression; dysthymic disorder.

Activity Intolerance
Related factors: Weakness/fatigue, Depression

Anxiety
Related factors: Change in role functioning, Change in interaction patterns, Threat to self-concept

Constipation
Related factors: Decreased activity, Medication (specify)

Coping, Ineffective Individual
Related factors: Personal vulnerability in situational crisis, Personal vulnerability in maturational crisis

Denial, Ineffective
Related factors: Specific to patient

Diversional Activity Deficit
Related factor: Disturbance in motivation

Family Processes, Altered
Related factor: Illness/disability of family member

Fatigue
Related factor: Overwhelming psychologic demands

Fear
Related factors: Real or imagined threat to own well-being, Powerlessness

Fluid Volume Deficit: High Risk
Risk factor: Deviations affecting access to or intake of fluids

Grieving, Dysfunctional
Related factors: Actual loss (specify), Anticipated loss (specify), Perceived loss (specify)

Health Maintenance, Altered
Related factors: Lack of ability to make deliberate and thoughtful judgments, Significant alteration in communication skills

Home Maintenance Management, Impaired
Related factor: Psychologic impairment (specify)

Hopelessness
Related factor: Long-term stress

Injury: High Risk
Risk factors: Psychologic: Affective factors, Orientation; Chemical: Drugs (alcohol, caffeine, nicotine); Physical: Cognitive, affective, and psychomotor factors

Nutrition, Altered: Less Than Body Requirements
Related factor: Psychologic impairment (specify)

Nutrition, Altered: More Than Body Requirements
Related factor: Psychologic impairment (specify)

Oral Mucous Membrane, Altered
Related factor: Medication (antidepressants)

Parenting, Altered
Related factor: Psychologic impairment (specify)

Personal Identity Disturbance
Related factor: Psychologic impairment (specify)

Post-Trauma Response
Related factors: Abuse, Accidents, Assault, Disaster, Epidemic, Incest, Kidnapping, Rape, Torture, Catastrophic illness or accident, Participation in combat

Powerlessness
Related factor: Psychologic impairment (specify)

Rape-Trauma Syndrome
Related factor: Biopsychosocial response by patient to event

Role Performance, Altered
Related factor: Psychologic impairment (specify)

Self-Care Deficit: Bathing/Hygiene, Dressing/Grooming, Feeding, Toileting (specify)
Related factor: Depression

Self-Esteem, Low: Chronic
Related factors: Psychologic impairment (specify), Repeatedly unmet expectations

Self-Mutilation: High Risk
Risk factors: Inability to cope with increased psychologic/physiologic tension in a healthy manner, Feelings of depression, rejection, self-hatred, separation anxiety, guilt, and depersonalization

Sexuality Patterns, Altered
Related factor: Disturbance in self-esteem

Sleep Pattern Disturbance
Related factors: Anxiety, Psychologic impairment (depression)

Social Interaction, Impaired
Related factor: Psychologic impairment (depression)

Thought Processes, Altered
Related factor: Mental disorder (specify)

Violence, High Risk: Self-Directed or Directed at Others
Risk factor: Suicidal ideation/intent

■ SUBSTANCE ABUSE PATIENT

Alcohol/drug intoxication/withdrawal/
dependence.

Anxiety
Related factors: Change in health status,
Change in role functioning, Situational
crisis, Unmet needs

Body Temperature, Altered: High Risk
Risk factor: Dehydration

Coping, Defensive
Related factor: Psychologic impairment
(substance abuse)

Coping, Ineffective Family: Compromised
Related factors: Temporary family
disorganization and role changes,
Unrealistic expectations/demands, Lack
of mutual decision-making skills,
Inadequate information/understanding
by family member

Coping, Ineffective Family: Disabling
Related factors: Arbitrary disregard for
patient's needs, Chronically unresolved
feelings (specify guilt, anxiety, hostility,
despair, etc.), Conflicting coping styles,
Highly ambivalent family relationships,
Violence used to manage conflict

Coping, Ineffective Individual
Related factors: Personal vulnerability in
situational crisis (specify), Personal
vulnerability in maturational crisis
(specify)

Decisional Conflict
Related factor: Chemical dependence

Denial, Ineffective
Related factors: Specific to patient

Diarrhea
Related factors: Excessive alcohol
intake, Excessive substance abuse

Fluid Volume Deficit: High Risk
Risk factor: Excessive, continuous
consumption of alcohol

Fluid Volume Excess
Related factor: Increased fluid intake
secondary to thirst

Grieving, Dysfunctional
Related factors: Actual loss (specify),
Anticipated loss (specify), Perceived loss
(specify)

Health Maintenance, Altered
Related factor: Lack of ability to make
deliberate and thoughtful judgments

Home Maintenance Management, Impaired
Related factors: Insufficient family
organization or planning, Psychologic
impairment (substance abuse)

Injury: High Risk
Risk factors: Psychologic: Affective
factors, Orientation; Chemical: Drugs
(alcohol, caffeine, nicotine)

Noncompliance
Related factors: Denial of illness,
Negative perception of treatment
regimen

Nutrition, Altered: Less Than Body Requirements
Related factor: Chemical dependence
(specify)

Pain, Chronic
Related factors: Specific to patient

Parenting, Altered
Related factors: Dysfunctional relationship between parents, Change in marital
status, Psychologic impairment (substance abuse)

Post-Trauma Response
Related factors: Abuse, Accidents,
Assault, Disaster, Epidemic, Incest,
Kidnapping, Rape, Torture, Terrorism,
Participation in combat

Powerlessness
Related factor: Pattern of helplessness

Rape-Trauma Syndrome
Related factor: Biopsychosocial response
of patient to event

Role Performance, Altered
Related factor: Psychologic impairment (substance abuse)

Self-Esteem, Low: Chronic
Related factor: Repeatedly unmet expectations

Self-Mutilation: High Risk
Risk factors: Inability to cope with increased psychologic/physiologic tension in a healthy manner, Drug/ alcohol abuse

Sensory/Perceptual Alterations: Visual, Auditory, Kinesthetic, Tactile
Related factors: Alcohol intoxication, Substance intoxication (specify)

Sexuality Patterns, Altered
Related factors: Disturbance in self-esteem, Substance abuse

Sleep Pattern Disturbance
Related factor: Chemical dependence (specify)

Social Interaction, Impaired
Related factor: Chemical dependence (specify)

Therapeutic Regimen Management, Ineffective Individual
Related factors: Decisional Conflict, Family patterns of health care, Inadequate number and types of cues to action, Knowledge deficit, Perceived seriousness, Perceived benefits, Powerlessness, Social support deficits

Violence, High Risk: Self-Directed or Directed at Others
Risk factors: Substance intoxication (specify), Substance withdrawal (specify)

■ SUICIDAL PATIENT

Associated psychiatric diagnoses include but are not limited to schizophrenia: disorganized type, catatonic type, paranoid type, undifferentiated type; schizophreniform disorder; affective disorders: manic episode, major depressive episode, bipolar disorders (mixed, manic, depressed), major depression (single episode, recurrent); panic disorders; post-traumatic stress disorder; organic mental disorders: primary degenerative dementia with depression, multi-infarct dementia with depression, alcohol/substance intoxication/ withdrawal/dependence; personality disorders: borderline personality disorder, schizoid personality disorder.

Anxiety
Related factors: Threat to self-concept, Threat to/change in role functioning, Situational/maturational crises, Unmet needs

Coping, Ineffective Family: Compromised
Related factors: Temporary family disorganization and role changes, Unrealistic expectations/demands, Lack of mutual decision-making skills, Inadequate understanding by family member

Coping, Ineffective Family: Disabling
Related factor: Highly ambivalent family relationships

Coping, Ineffective Individual
Related factors: Personal vulnerability in situational crisis (specify), Personal vulnerability in maturational crisis (specify)

Decisional Conflict
Related factors: Perceived threat to value system, Lack of support system

Denial, Ineffective
Related factors: Specific to patient

Fear
Related factors: Powerlessness, Real or imagined threat to own well-being

Hopelessness
Related factors: Abandonment, Lack of social supports, Lost spiritual belief

Personal Identity Disturbance
Related factor: Situational crisis
(specify)

Post-Trauma Response
Related factors: Abuse, Accidents,
Assault, Disaster, Epidemic, Incest,
Kidnapping, Rape, Terrorism, Torture,
Catastrophic illness or accident, Partici-
pation in combat

Rape-Trauma Syndrome
Related factor: Patient's biopsychosocial
response to event

Role Performance, Altered
Related factors: Situational crisis
(specify), Psychologic impairment
(specify)

Self-Esteem, Low: Chronic
Related factors: Psychologic impairment (specify), Repeatedly unmet
expectations

Self-Esteem, Low: Situational
Related factor: Situational crisis
(specify)

Self-Mutilation: High Risk
Risk factors: Inability to cope with
increased psychologic/physiologic
tension in a healthy manner, Feelings of
depression, rejection, self-hatred,
separation anxiety, guilt, and
depersonalization, Fluctuating emotions,
Drug/alcohol abuse

**Sensory/Perceptual Alterations: Visual,
Auditory, Kinesthetic, Gustatory,
Tactile, Olfactory (specify)**
Related factor: Alcohol/substance abuse
(specify)

Thought Processes, Altered
Related factors: Mental disorder
(specify), Organic mental disorder
(specify), Personality disorder (specify),
Substance abuse

**Violence, High Risk: Self-Directed or
Directed at Others**
Risk factors: History of suicide attempt,
Command hallucinations, Battered
women, Panic states, History of abuse
by others, Suicidal ideation, Substance
abuse

■ WITHDRAWN PATIENT

Associated psychiatric diagnoses include but
are not limited to major depression; schizophrenia: disorganized type, catatonic type,
paranoid type, undifferentiated type;
schizophreniform disorder; phobic disorders;
schizoid personality disorder; avoidant
personality disorder; substance abuse
disorders; organic mental disorders.

Anxiety
Related factors: Threat to role functioning, Change in role functioning

Communication, Impaired: Verbal
Related factor: Psychologic impairment
(specify)

Coping, Ineffective Individual
Related factors: Personal vulnerability in
situational crisis (specify), Personal
vulnerability in maturational crisis
(specify)

Denial, Ineffective
Related factors: Specific to patient

Diversional Activity Deficit
Related factors: Disturbance in motivation, Deficit in social skills, Impaired
perception of reality

Family Processes, Altered
Related factor: Illness/disability of
family member

Fear
Related factors: Powerlessness, Real or
imagined threat to own well-being

Grieving, Dysfunctional
Related factors: Actual loss (specify),
Anticipated loss (specify), Perceived loss
(specify)

Health Maintenance, Altered
Related factors: Lack of ability to make
thoughtful and deliberate judgments,
Significant alteration in communication
skills

Hopelessness
Related factors: Lack of social supports,
Long-term stress

Parenting, Altered
Related factors: Psychologic impairment
(specify), Situational crisis (specify)

Post-Trauma Response
Related factors: Abuse, Accidents,
Assault, Disaster, Epidemic, Incest,
Kidnapping, Rape, Terrorism, Torture,
Catastrophic illness or event, Participa-
tion in combat

Rape-Trauma Syndrome: Silent reaction
Related factor: Patient's biopsychosocial
response to event

Role Performance, Altered
Related factors: Psychologic impairment
(specify)

Self-Esteem, Low: Chronic
Related factors: Psychologic impairment (specify), Repeatedly unmet
expectations

Self-Esteem, Low: Situational
Related factor: Situational crisis

Self-Mutilation: High Risk
Risk factors: Inability to cope with
increased psychologic/physiologic
tension in a healthy manner, Feelings of
depression, rejection, self-hatred,
separation anxiety, guilt, and
depersonalization, Need for sensory
stimuli

Sleep Pattern Disturbance
Related factor: Psychologic impairment
(specify)

Social Interaction, Impaired
Related factor: Psychologic impairment
(specify)

Social Isolation
Related factor: Psychologic impairment
(specify)

Thought Processes, Altered
Related factors: Mental disorder
(specify), Organic mental disorder
(specify), Personality disorder (specify)

Antepartum and Postpartum Conditions

Abortion, induced or elective
Change in birthing plans
Gestational diabetes
Hyperemesis gravidarum
Maternal infection
Painful breast
Perinatal loss

Postpartum care,
   Uncomplicated
Pregnancy-induced
   hypertension
Suppression of preterm labor
Uterine bleeding

■ ABORTION, INDUCED OR ELECTIVE

Coping, Ineffective Individual
Related factor: Unresolved feelings about elective abortion

Fluid Volume Deficit
Related factor: Abnormal blood loss secondary to incomplete abortion

Infection: High Risk
Risk factors: Invasive procedures, Broken skin, Traumatized tissue

Knowledge Deficit (specify)
Related factor: Limited exposure to information (contraception)

Pain [Acute]
Related factor: Strong uterine contractions

Powerlessness
Related factor: Treatment regimen

Self-Esteem Disturbance
Related factors: Unmet expectations for pregnancy, Unmet expectations for child

Sexual Dysfunction
Related factor: Disturbance in self-esteem

Spiritual Distress
Related factor: Test of spiritual beliefs

■ CHANGE IN BIRTHING PLANS

May include any deviation from a couple's original birthing plans. Includes but is not limited to use of analgesia, anesthesia, or forceps, limitation of visitors, episiotomy, cesarean birth.

Body Image Disturbance
Related factor: Surgery

Family Processes, Altered,
Related factor: Unmet expectations for childbirth

Fear
Related factors: Real or imagined threat to child, Real or imagined threat to own well-being

Knowledge Deficit (specify)
Related factor: Limited exposure to information

Pain [Acute]
Related factors: Surgery, Episiotomy

Powerlessness
Related factor: Complication threatening pregnancy

Role Performance, Altered
Related factor: Unmet expectations for childbirth

Self-Esteem Disturbance
Related factor: Unmet expectations for childbirth

■ GESTATIONAL DIABETES

Family Processes, Altered
Related factors: Hospitalization/change in environment, Illness/disability of family member

Fear
Related factors: Environmental stressors/hospitalization, Powerlessness, Real or imagined threat to own well-being, Real or imagined threat to child, Implications for future pregnancies

Injury: High Risk (Maternal or Fetal)
Risk factors: Hypoglycemia, Hyperglycemia

Knowledge Deficit (specify)
Related factors: Limited exposure to information (specify), Preparation for childbirth, Signs and symptoms of premature labor, Premature rupture of membranes, Blood glucose testing, Insulin dosage and administration

Nutrition, Altered: Less Than Body Requirements
Related factor: Limited exposure to new basic nutritional knowledge

Nutrition, Altered: More Than Body Requirements
Related factor: Limited exposure to new basic nutritional knowledge

Self-Esteem Disturbance
Related factor: Unmet expectations for pregnancy

Therapeutic Regimen Management, Ineffective Individual
Related factors: Complexity of therapeutic regimen, Knowledge deficits, Perceived seriousness, Social supports deficits

■ HYPEREMESIS GRAVIDARUM

Coping, Ineffective Individual
Related factor: Personal vulnerability during health crisis

Family Processes, Altered
Related factors: Hospitalization/change in environment, Illness/disability of family member

Fatigue
Related factor: Disease process

Fear
Related factor: Real or imagined threat to child

Fluid Volume Deficit
Related factors: Inadequate fluid intake, Abnormal fluid loss secondary to vomiting

Knowledge Deficit (specify)
Related factor: Limited exposure to information (specify)

Nutrition, Altered: Less Than Body Requirements
Related factor: Nausea and/or vomiting

Powerlessness
Related factor: Complications threatening pregnancy

Role Performance, Altered
Related factor: Unmet expectations for pregnancy

Self-Esteem Disturbance
Related factor: Unmet expectations for pregnancy

■ MATERNAL INFECTION

Includes but is not limited to active genital herpes, amnionitis, acquired immune deficiency syndrome, hepatitis B.

Body Image Disturbance
Related factors: Pregnancy, Infection

Breast-Feeding, Interrupted
Related factors: Maternal illness, Maternal medications that are contraindicated for the infant

Family Processes, Altered
Related factors: Change in family roles, Hospitalization/change in environment

Fatigue
Related factor: Disease process

Fear
Related factor: Real or imagined threat to child

Knowledge Deficit (specify)
Related factor: Limited exposure to information (specify)

Pain [Acute]
Related factors: Cesarean birth, Infection

Parenting, Altered: High Risk
Risk factor: Delayed parent/infant attachment

Self-Esteem Disturbance
Related factors: Cesarean birth, Assumption of new role

Social Interaction, Impaired
Related factor: Therapeutic isolation

Social Isolation
Related factor: Medical condition (specify)

■ PAINFUL BREAST

Includes but is not limited to sore, cracked nipples, engorgement, mastitis.

Breast-Feeding, Ineffective
Related factor: Breast pain

Breast-Feeding, Interrupted
Related factors: Engorgement, Sore, cracked nipples, Mastitis, Maternal medications that are contraindicated for the infant

Knowledge Deficit (specify)
Related factors: Limited exposure to information about breast hygiene, Limited exposure to information about care of nipples, Limited exposure to information about signs and symptoms of infection

Pain [Acute]
Related factors: Sore nipples, Breast engorgement, Infection

Role Performance, Altered
Related factors: Assumption of new role, Unmet expectations for childbirth

Self-Esteem Disturbance
Related factor: Unmet expectations for childbirth

Skin Integrity, Impaired: High Risk
Risk factors: Inadequate breast care, Breast-feeding

■ PERINATAL LOSS

Includes but is not limited to less than perfect baby, miscarriage, stillbirth, adoption, elective abortion.

Coping, Ineffective Family: Disabling
Related factor: Chronically unresolved feelings about loss

Coping, Ineffective Individual
Related factor: Personal vulnerability in a situational crisis

Family Processes, Altered
Related factors: Illness/disability of baby, Lack of adequate support system

Fear
Related factors: Real or imagined threat to child, Environmental stressors/ hospitalization, Powerlessness, Implications for future pregnancies

Grieving, Anticipatory
Related factors: Imminent loss of child, Anticipated loss of perfect child

Grieving, Dysfunctional
Related factors: Actual or anticipated loss of child, Actual or anticipated loss of perfect child

Knowledge Deficit (specify)
Related factors: Limited exposure to information (specify), Limited practice of skill (specify), Information misinterpretation

Parenting, Altered
Related factors: Interruption in bonding process, Unrealistic expectations of self or partner

Powerlessness
Related factor: Complication threatening pregnancy

Role Performance, Altered
Related factors: Loss of child, Birth of less than perfect baby

Self-Esteem Disturbance
Related factor: Unmet expectations for child

Sexual Dysfunction
Related factors: Medically imposed restrictions, Fear of harming fetus, Disturbance in self-esteem

Spiritual Distress
Related factor: Test of spiritual beliefs

■ POSTPARTUM CARE, UNCOMPLICATED

Activity Intolerance
Related factor: Weakness/fatigue

Anxiety
Related factor: Change in role functioning

Body Image Disturbance
Related factor: Lack of or inaccurate information about body's adjustment after delivery

Breast-Feeding, Effective (Potential for Enhanced)
Related factors: Basic breast-feeding knowledge, Normal breast structure, Normal infant oral structure, Gestational age of more than 34 weeks, Supportive resources, Maternal confidence

Constipation
Related factors: Painful defecation, Decreased activity, Decreased fluid intake

Coping, Ineffective Individual
Related factor: Personal vulnerability in a maturational crisis

Family Processes, Altered
Related factors: Change in family roles, Change in family structure, Lack of adequate support systems

Fatigue
Related factors: Excessive social demands and/or role demands, Pain

Fluid Volume Deficit
Related factors: Abnormal fluid loss secondary to diuresis, Decreased fluid intake

Home Maintenance Management, Impaired
Related factor: Inadequate support system

Infection: High Risk
Risk factors: Broken skin, Traumatized tissue, Invasive procedures

Knowledge Deficit (specify)
Related factor: Lack of exposure to information about self-care, baby care, bonding, family-planning methods, infant growth and development

Nutrition, Altered: Less Than Body Requirements
Related factor: Lack of basic nutritional knowledge concerning lactation

Pain [Acute]
Related factors: Pain secondary to episiotomy, Sore nipples, Breast engorgement, Hemorrhoids, Spinal headache

Parenting, Altered: High Risk
Risk factors: Lack of knowledge/skill regarding effective parenting, Unrealistic expectations of self, infant, partner

Role Performance, Altered
Related factor: Assumption of new role

Sexual Dysfunction
Related factors: Pain, Recent childbirth, Disturbance in self-esteem

■ PREGNANCY-INDUCED HYPERTENSION

Also known as toxemia of pregnancy, preeclampsia, eclampsia

Activity Intolerance
Related factors: Imbalance between oxygen supply and demand, Weakness/fatigue

Body Image Disturbance
Related factors: Pregnancy and edema

Cardiac Output, Decreased
Related factor: Increased ventricular workload

Diversional Activity Deficit
Related factor: Prolonged bed rest

Family Processes, Altered
Related factors: Hospitalization/change in environment, Illness/disability of family member

Fatigue
Related factor: Disease process

Fear
Related factors: Changes in birthing plans, Real or imagined threat to child, Environmental stressors/hospitalization, Real or imagined threat to own well-being, Implications for future pregnancies

Fluid Volume Excess
Related factors: Sodium and water retention

Home Maintenance Management, Impaired
Related factor: Inadequate support system

Injury: High Risk (Maternal and Fetal)
Risk factors: Seizure activity, Inadequate placental perfusion

Knowledge Deficit (specify)
Related factor: Limited exposure to information (specify)

Mobility, Impaired Physical
Related factor: Medically prescribed limitations

Nutrition, Altered: Less Than Body Requirements
Related factors: Lack of basic nutritional knowledge, Loss of appetite, Nausea/vomiting

Powerlessness
Related factor: Complications threatening pregnancy

Therapeutic Regimen Management, Ineffective Individual
Related factors: Knowledge deficits, Perceived seriousness, Perceived benefits

Tissue Perfusion, Altered: Cerebral, Renal, Placental
Related factors: Vasospasm, Edema, Decreased intravascular volume

■ SUPPRESSION OF PRETERM LABOR

Anxiety
Related factor: Outcome of pregnancy

Coping, Ineffective Individual
Related factor: Personal vulnerability in situational crisis

Diversional Activity Deficit
Related factor: Prolonged bed rest

Family Processes, Altered
Related factors: Illness/disability of family member, Change in family roles, Lack of adequate support systems

Fear
Related factor: Possibility of early labor and delivery

Home Maintenance Management, Impaired
Related factor: Inadequate support system

Knowledge Deficit (specify)
Related factor: Limited exposure to information re causes, identification, and treatment of preterm labor

Powerlessness
Related factor: Complications threatening pregnancy

Self-Care Deficit: Bathing/Hygiene, Dressing/Grooming, Feeding, Toileting (specify)
Related factor: Medically imposed restrictions

Self-Esteem Disturbance
Related factor: Unmet expectations for childbirth

Sexual Dysfunction
Related factors: Medically imposed restrictions, Fear of harming fetus

Sleep Pattern Disturbance
Related factors: Frequency of medication and monitoring

Therapeutic Regimen Management, Ineffective Individual
Related factors: Knowledge deficits, Excessive demands made on individual/family, Social support deficits

■ UTERINE BLEEDING

Includes but is not limited to the following: *Antepartal:* first trimester spotting, placenta previa, abruptio placentae, uterine rupture, hydatidiform mole. *Postpartal:* postpartum hemorrhage/shock; uterine atony.

Breast-Feeding, Interrupted
Related factors: Maternal illness, Fatigue

Cardiac Output, Decreased
Related factor: Hypovolemia

Constipation
Related factor: Decreased activity

Diversional Activity Deficit
Related factor: Prolonged bed rest

Family Processes, Altered
Related factors: Change in family roles, Hospitalization/change in environment, Illness/disability of family member

Fear
Related factors: Real or imagined threat to child, Real or imagined threat to own well-being, Powerlessness, Environmental stressors/hospitalization, Implications for future pregnancies

Fluid Volume Deficit
Related factor: Abnormal blood loss

Home Maintenance Management, Impaired
Related factor: Inadequate support system

Infection: High Risk
Risk factors: Traumatized tissue, Invasive procedures

Knowledge Deficit (specify)
Related factor: Limited exposure to information re recovery

Pain [Acute]
Related factors: Nausea and/or vomiting, Surgical procedure, Uterine contractions

Powerlessness
Related factor: Complications threatening pregnancy

Self-Care Deficit: Bathing/Hygiene, Dressing/Grooming, Feeding, Toileting (specify)
Related factor: Medically imposed restrictions

Self-Esteem Disturbance
Related factor: Unmet expectations for childbirth

Sexual Dysfunction
Related factors: Medically imposed restrictions, Fear of harming fetus

Therapeutic Regimen Management, Ineffective Individual
Related factors: Knowledge deficits, Excessive demands made on individual/family, Social support deficits

Tissue Perfusion, Altered: Placental
Related factor: Imbalance between oxygen supply/demand to the fetus secondary to hypovolemia, hypotension, placental separation

Newborn Conditions

Bleeding/obstruction of urinary
   tract postcircumcision
Drug withdrawal
Feeding problems
High-risk infant
Hyperbilirubinemia

Hypoglycemia
Hypothermia
Inability to adapt to
   extrauterine life
Low birth weight
Respiratory distress

■ BLEEDING/OBSTRUCTION OF
URINARY TRACT POSTCIRCUMCISION

Fluid Volume Deficit
Related factor: Abnormal blood loss

Pain [Acute]
Related factor: Surgery

Urinary Retention
Related factor: Urethral obstruction

■ DRUG WITHDRAWAL

Breast-Feeding, Ineffective
Related factor: Infant fatigue

Breathing Pattern, Ineffective
Related factor: Depression of respiratory center secondary to ___ (specify drug)

Coping, Ineffective Family: Disabling
Related factor: Arbitrary disregard for patient's needs

Fluid Volume Deficit
Related factor: Inadequate fluid intake secondary to inadequate suckling reflex

Growth and Development, Altered
Related factor: Unhealthy maternal lifestyle during pregnancy

Home Maintenance Management, Impaired
Related factors: Physical/psychologic impairment of family member other than patient, Inadequate support system, Insufficient family organization or planning

Infant Feeding Pattern, Ineffective
Related factor: Neurological impairment/delay

Injury: High Risk
Risk factors: Psychomotor hyperactivity, Seizure activity

Nutrition, Altered: Less Than Body Requirements
Related factors: Chemical dependence, Inadequate sucking reflex in infant, Vomiting, Food intolerance

Parenting, Altered
Related factors: Psychologic impairment, Substance abuse

Sleep Pattern Disturbance
Related factors: Sleep deprivation secondary to ___ (specify), Effect of depressants or stimulants

■ FEEDING PROBLEMS

Include but are not limited to the infant with food allergies or intolerances, malabsorption, or abnormal motor problems that affect the infant's ability to consume food.

Breast-Feeding, Ineffective
Related factors: Inadequate sucking reflex in infant, Infant fatigue, Inability of infant to "latch on"

Constipation
Related factor: Decreased fluid intake

Diarrhea
Related factor: Food intolerance

Family Processes, Altered
Related factors: Illness/disability of family member, Separation of family members

Fluid Volume Deficit
Related factor: Inadequate fluid intake

Infant Feeding Pattern, Ineffective
Related factors: Prematurity, Neurological impairment/delay, Oral hypersensitivity, Prolonged NPO, Anatomical abnormalities

Nutrition, Altered: Less Than Body Requirements
Related factors: Difficulty in swallowing, Inadequate sucking reflex in the infant, Vomiting, Food intolerance

Swallowing, Impaired
Related factor: Abnormal motor problem (specify)

■ HIGH-RISK INFANT

Includes but is not limited to birth asphyxia, meconium aspiration, prematurity, premature rupture of membranes, maternal infection, infant of diabetic mother, intrauterine growth retardation, infant of adolescent mother, infant of chemically dependent mother, lack of prenatal care.

Airway Clearance, Ineffective
Related factors: Meconium aspiration, Tracheobronchial secretions

Aspiration: High Risk
Risk factor: Presence of enteral or tracheal tubes

Body Temperature, Altered: High Risk
Risk factor: Immaturity of newborn's temperature-regulating system

Breast-Feeding, Ineffective
Related factors: Infant fatigue, Inadequate sucking reflex, Interrupted or infrequent feeding

Breast-Feeding, Interrupted
Related factors: Infant illness, Prematurity, Maternal obligations outside the home, Abrupt weaning of infant

Breathing Pattern, Ineffective
Related factor: Decreased energy/fatigue

Cardiac Output, Decreased
Related factors: Increased ventricular workload, Hypovolemia, Cardiac anomaly (specify)

Caregiver Role Strain (Actual/High Risk)
Related factors/risk factors: Illness severity of the care receiver, Premature birth/congenital defect, Unpredictable illness course, Situational stressors within the family, Chronicity of caregiving, Caregiver's health, developmental readiness, knowledge, skills, experience, competing role commitments, coping styles, isolation, opportunity for respite and recreation

Diarrhea
Related factor: Increased intestinal motility secondary to inflammation

Dysfunctional Ventilatory Weaning Response (DVWR)
Related factors: Pulmonary immaturity, Impaired gas exchange, Ineffective airway clearance, Ventilator dependence >1 week

Family Processes, Altered
Related factors: Illness/disability of family member, Separation of family members

Fatigue
Related factor: Disease process

Fear (Parental)
Related factor: Threat to child

Fluid Volume Deficit
Related factors: Abnormal blood loss, Abnormal fluid loss (specify), Inadequate fluid intake secondary to ___ (specify)

Fluid Volume Excess
Related factor: Decreased urinary output secondary to heart failure

Gas Exchange, Impaired
Related factor: Decreased functional lung tissue secondary to pneumonia, chronic lung disease, atelectasis

Grieving, Anticipatory (Parental)
Related factor: Imminent loss of child

Growth and Development, Altered
Related factors: Congenital anomaly, Fetal distress, Prematurity, Unhealthy maternal life-style during pregnancy, Serious illness

Home Maintenance Management, Impaired
Related factors: Inadequate support system, Insufficient family organization or planning

Infant Feeding Pattern, Ineffective
Related factors: Prematurity, Neurological impairment/delay, Prolonged NPO, Anatomical abnormalities

Infection: High Risk
Risk factors: Inadequate immune system, Insufficient family organization or planning

Nutrition, Altered: Less Than Body Requirements
Related factors: Inadequate sucking reflex in the infant, Vomiting, Food intolerance, High metabolic states

Spontaneous Ventilation, Inability to Sustain
Related factors: Metabolic factors, Respiratory muscle fatigue, Pulmonary immaturity

■ HYPERBILIRUBINEMIA

Breast-Feeding, Interrupted
Related factor: Infant illness

Diarrhea
Related factor: Dietary changes

Family Processes, Altered
Related factor: Separation of family members

Fluid Volume Deficit
Related factors: Abnormal fluid loss (specify), Inadequate fluid intake secondary to ___ (specify)

Nutrition, Altered: Less Than Body Requirements
Related factors: Lethargy, Inadequate sucking reflex in infant

Parenting, Altered
Related factor: Interruption in bonding process

Sensory/Perceptual Alterations: Visual
Related factor: Sensory deficit secondary to use of eye patches for protection of eyes during phototherapy

Skin Integrity, Impaired: High Risk
Risk factors: Incontinence of stool, Drying of skin secondary to phototherapy, Pruritus

Sleep Pattern Disturbance
Related factor: Sleep deprivation

■ HYPOGLYCEMIA

Cardiac Output, Decreased
Related factor: Poor cardiac contractility

Family Processes, Altered
Related factors: Illness/disability of family member, Separation of family members

Injury: High Risk
Risk factor: Seizure activity

Nutrition, Altered: Less Than Body Requirements
Related factors: Inadequate sucking reflex in infant, High metabolic states/physiologic stress

■ HYPOTHERMIA

Breathing Pattern, Ineffective
Related factor: Decreased energy/fatigue

Cardiac Output, Decreased
Related factor: Bradycardia

Family Processes, Altered
Related factor: Separation of family members

Nutrition, Altered: Less Than Body Requirements
Related factor: Loss of/decreased appetite

Tissue Perfusion, Altered: Peripheral
Related factor: Imbalance between oxygen supply/demand

■ INABILITY TO ADAPT TO EXTRAUTERINE LIFE

Includes but is not limited to premature infants and infants with serious congenital anomalies.

Activity Intolerance
Related factor: Imbalance between oxygen supply and demand

Body Temperature, Altered: High Risk
Risk factor: Immaturity of newborn's temperature-regulating system

Breast-Feeding, Ineffective
Related factors: Infant fatigue, Inadequate sucking reflex, Interrupted or infrequent feeding

Breathing Pattern, Ineffective
Related factor: Decreased energy/fatigue

Cardiac Output, Decreased
Related factors: Increased ventricular workload, Hypovolemia, Cardiac anomaly (specify)

Caregiver Role Strain (Actual/High Risk)
Related factors/risk factors: Illness severity of the care receiver, Premature birth/congenital defect, Unpredictable illness course, Situational stressors within the family, Chronicity of caregiving, Caregiver's health, developmental readiness, knowledge, skills, experience, competing role commitments, coping styles, isolation, opportunity for respite and recreation

Dysfunctional Ventilatory Weaning Response (DVWR)
Related factors: Pulmonary immaturity, Impaired gas exchange, Ineffective airway clearance, Ventilator dependence > 1 week

Family Processes, Altered
Related factors: Unmet expectations for child, Separation of family members, Illness/disability of family member

Fatigue
Related factor: Disease process

Fear
Related factor: Real threat to child

Fluid Volume Deficit
Related factors: Abnormal blood loss, Abnormal fluid loss (specify), Inadequate fluid intake secondary to ___ (specify)

Gas Exchange, Impaired
Related factors: Decreased pulmonary blood supply secondary to pulmonary hypertension, congestive heart failure, respiratory distress syndrome, Decreased functional lung tissue secondary to respiratory distress syndrome, atelectasis

Grieving, Anticipatory
Related factor: Anticipatory loss of child

Growth and Development, Altered
Related factors: Congenital anomaly, Fetal distress, Prematurity, Unhealthy maternal life-style during pregnancy, Serious illness

Infant Feeding Pattern, Ineffective
Related factors: Prematurity, Neurological impairment/delay, Prolonged NPO, Anatomical abnormalities

Nutrition, Altered: Less Than Body Requirements
Related factors: Difficulty in swallowing, Inadequate sucking reflex in infant, Vomiting, Food intolerance

Skin Integrity, Impaired: High Risk
Risk factors: Impaired circulation, Immobility, Altered nutritional status

Sleep Pattern Disturbance
Related factor: Sleep deprivation secondary to frequent therapeutic interventions

Spontaneous Ventilation, Inability to Sustain
Related factors: Metabolic factors, Respiratory muscle fatigue, Pulmonary immaturity

Tissue Perfusion, Altered: Peripheral
Related factor: Imbalance between oxygen supply/demand secondary to high metabolic state

Urinary Retention
Related factor: Congenital anomaly (specify)

■ LOW BIRTH WEIGHT

Activity Intolerance
Related factor: Weakness/fatigue

Airway Clearance, Ineffective
Related factors: Decreased energy/
fatigue

Body Temperature, Altered: High Risk
Risk factor: Immaturity of newborn's
temperature-regulating system

Breast-Feeding, Ineffective
Related factors: Infant fatigue, Inadequate sucking reflex, Interrupted or
infrequent feeding

Breast-Feeding, Interrupted
Related factor: Prematurity

Breathing Pattern, Ineffective
Related factor: Decreased energy/fatigue

Constipation
Related factor: Decreased fluid intake

Family Processes, Altered
Related factors: Illness/disablity of
family member, Separation of family
members

Fatigue
Related factor: Decreased energy

Fluid Volume Deficit
Related factor: Inadequate fluid intake

Gas Exchange, Impaired
Related factors: Decreased pulmonary
blood supply secondary to respiratory
distress syndrome, Decreased functional
lung tissue secondary to atelectasis,
respiratory distress syndrome

Grieving, Dysfunctional
Related factor: Anticipated or perceived
loss of the perfect child

**Home Maintenance Management,
Impaired**
Related factors: Inadequate support
system, Insufficient family organization
or planning

Infant Feeding Pattern, Ineffective
Related factor: Prematurity

**Nutrition, Altered: Less Than Body
Requirements**
Related factors: Inadequate sucking
reflex in infant, Food intolerance, High
metabolic state

Skin Integrity, Impaired: High Risk
Risk factors: Fragile skin, Lack of
subcutaneous fat

Sleep Pattern Disturbance
Related factor: Sleep deprivation
secondary to frequent therapeutic
interventions

**Spontaneous Ventilation, Inability to
Sustain**
Related factors: Metabolic factors,
Respiratory muscle fatigue, Pulmonary
immaturity

Tissue Perfusion, Altered: Peripheral
Related factor: Imbalance between
oxygen supply/demand

■ RESPIRATORY DISTRESS

Includes but is not limited to bronchopulmonary dysplasia, respiratory distress
syndrome/hyaline membrane disease,
meconium aspiration, pneumonia,
pneumothorax, transient tachypnea.

Activity Intolerance
Related factor: Weakness/fatigue

Airway Clearance, Ineffective
Related factors: Decreased energy/
fatigue, Tracheobronchial secretions

Aspiration: High Risk
Risk factor: Presence of enteral or
tracheal tubes

Breast-Feeding, Interrupted
Related factors: Prematurity, Infant
illness

Breathing Pattern, Ineffective
Related factors: Decreased energy/
fatigue, Dependence on ventilator

Cardiac Output, Decreased
Related factors: Increased ventricular workload, Cardiac anomaly (specify)

Caregiver Role Strain (Actual/High Risk)
Related factors/risk factors: Illness severity of the care receiver, Premature birth/congenital defect, Unpredictable illness course, Situational stressors within the family, Chronicity of caregiving, Caregiver's health, developmental readiness, knowledge, skills, experience, competing role commitments, coping styles, isolation, opportunity for respite and recreation

Constipation
Related factor: Decreased fluid intake

Dysfunctional Ventilatory Weaning Response (DVWR)
Related factors: Pulmonary immaturity, Impaired gas exchange, Ineffective airway clearance, Ventilator dependence >1 week

Family Processes, Altered
Related factors: Illness/disability of family member, Separation of family members

Fatigue
Related factor: Disease process

Fear (Parental)
Related factor: Real threat to child

Fluid Volume Deficit
Related factors: Inadequate fluid intake secondary to fatigue with oral feedings, Abnormal fluid loss (insensible water loss secondary to rapid respiratory rate)

Gas Exchange, Impaired
Related factors: Decreased pulmonary blood supply secondary to pulmonary hypertension/persistent fetal circulation, respiratory distress syndrome, Decreased functional lung tissue secondary to pneumonia, atelectasis, respiratory distress syndrome, Diaphragmatic hernia

Grieving, Anticipatory (Parental)
Related factor: Anticipated or perceived loss of child

Home Maintenance Management, Impaired
Related factors: Inadequate support system, Insufficient family planning or organization

Infant Feeding Pattern, Ineffective
Related factors: Prematurity, Anatomical abnormalities

Infection: High Risk
Risk factors: Inadequate immune system, Invasive monitoring

Nutrition, Altered: Less Than Body Requirements
Related factors: Inadequate sucking reflex in infant, Food intolerance, High metabolic state, Lethargy

Skin Integrity, Impaired: High Risk
Risk factor: Decreased peripheral perfusion

Sleep Pattern Disturbance
Related factor: Sleep deprivation secondary to frequent therapeutic interventions

Spontaneous Ventilation, Inability to Sustain
Related factors: Metabolic factors, Respiratory muscle fatigue, Pulmonary immaturity

Tissue Perfusion, Altered: Peripheral
Related factor: Imbalance between oxygen supply/demand

Pediatric Conditions

Burns
Cancer, see *Medical Conditions:* Cancer, pp. 249–250
Casts and traction
Child abuse
Chronic illness: Developmental problems/needs
Cleft lip/cleft palate: Surgical repair
Coagulation disorders
Congenital malformations of the central nervous system: Surgical repair
Diabetes mellitus, see *Medical Conditions:* Endocrine disorders, pp. 253–254
Failure to thrive
Gastroenteritis
Gastrointestinal obstruction: Surgical repair
Infection of central nervous system
Ingestion/accidental poisoning
Juvenile rheumatoid arthritis, see *Medical Conditions:* Arthritis, pp. 245–246

Obese child
Osteomyelitis
Pregnancy in adolescence
Renal failure, Acute, see *Medical Conditions:* Renal failure, Acute, p. 261
Renal failure, Chronic, see *Medical Conditions:* Renal failure, Chronic, pp. 261–263
Respiratory disorder, Chronic
Respiratory infection, Acute
Rheumatic fever, see *Medical Conditions:* Pericarditis/endocarditis, p. 259–260
Seizure disorders
Sepsis
Sickle cell crisis
Suicidal adolescent, see *Psychiatric Conditions:* Suicidal patient, pp. 290–291
Tonsillectomy

■ BURNS

Activity Intolerance
Related factor: Acute pain

Body Image Disturbance
Related factor: Burns

Body Temperature, Altered: High Risk
Risk factor: Dehydration secondary to
impairment in skin integrity

Constipation
Related factors: Decreased gastrointestinal motility, Dehydration

Coping, Ineffective Individual
Related factor: Severe injury

Diversional Activity Deficit
Related factors: Long-term hospitalization, Prolonged bed rest

Family Processes, Altered
Related factors: Hospitalization/change
in environment, Illness/disability of
family member

Fear
Related factors: Painful therapeutic
procedures, Environmental stressors/
hospitalization, Real threat to own
well-being

Fluid Volume Deficit
Related factor: Abnormal fluid loss
secondary to loss of skin integrity

**Home Maintenance Management,
Impaired**
Related factor: Lack of knowledge
concerning prevention of future burns

Infection: High Risk
Risk factors: Malnutrition, Broken skin

**Nutrition, Altered: Less Than Body
Requirements**
Related factor: High metabolic needs

Pain [Acute]
Related factor: Injury

Parental Role Conflict
Related factor: Intimidation with
invasive or restrictive modalities

**Self-Care Deficit: Bathing/Hygiene,
Dressing/Grooming, Feeding,
Toileting (specify)**
Related factor: Pain with movement

Skin Integrity, Impaired
Related factor: Burns

Social Interaction, Impaired
Related factors: Self-concept disturbance, Limited physical mobility

■ CASTS AND TRACTION

Includes but is not limited to orthopedic
trauma, congenital hip dysplasia.

Body Image Disturbance
Related factors: Surgery, Congenital
defects

Diversional Activity Deficit
Related factors: Forced inactivity,
Prolonged bed rest, Long-term
hospitalization

Family Processes, Altered
Related factors: Hospitalization/change
in environment, Illness/disability of
family member

Fear
Related factors: Environmental
stressors/hospitalization

Infection: High Risk
Risk factors: Trauma, Broken skin

Mobility, Impaired Physical
Related factors: Pain/discomfort,
Medically imposed restrictions, Muscu-
loskeletal impairment

Pain [Acute]
Related factors: Pain secondary to
injury, Pain secondary to surgery,
Pruritus, Paresthesia

Peripheral Neurovascular Dysfunction
Related factor: Immobilization

**Self-Care Deficit: Bathing/Hygiene,
Dressing/Grooming, Feeding,
Toileting (specify)**
Related factors: Pain/discomfort,
Musculoskeletal impairment, Medically
imposed restrictions

Skin Integrity: High Risk
Risk factors: Altered circulation,
Physical immobilization

Tissue Perfusion, Altered: Peripheral
Related factors: Interruption of venous
flow to ___ (specify) secondary to
constriction pressure, Interruption of
arterial flow to ___ (specify) secondary
to compartment syndrome

Urinary Incontinence, Functional
Related factor: Mobility deficits

■ CHILD ABUSE

Caregiver Role Strain (Actual)
Related factor: Presence of abuse or
violence

Coping, Ineffective Family: Disabling
Related factors: Chronically unresolved
feelings (specify), Highly ambivalent
family relationships, Substance-abusing
family member, Emotionally disturbed
family member, Use of violence to
manage conflict, Child sexual/physical
abuse

Coping, Ineffective Individual
Related factor: Personal vulnerability in
situational crisis

Fear
Related factors: Real threat to own well-
being, Powerlessness

Growth and Development, Altered
Related factor: Abuse

**Home Maintenance Management,
Impaired**
Related factors: Physical/psychologic
impairment of family member other
than patient, Inadequate support
system, Developmental disability,
Psychologic impairment, Lack of
knowledge

Hopelessness
Related factor: Long-term stress

Injury: High Risk
Risk factors: Physical/psychologic abuse,
Parental neglect

Knowledge Deficit (specify)
Related factors: Limited exposure to
information about normal growth and
development of children, Limited
practice of parenting skills, Cognitive
limitations

**Nutrition, Altered: Less Than Body
Requirements**
Related factor: Parental neglect

Pain [Acute]
Related factor: Trauma

Parental Role Conflict
Related factors: Change in marital
status, Relocation, Financial or legal
crisis

Parenting, Altered
Related factors: Absent or ineffective
role model, Interruption in bonding
process, Lack of knowledge/skill, Lack
of or inappropriate response of child to
parent, Lack of support for nurturing
figure(s), Psychologic impairment;
Physical illness, Unrealistic expectations
of self, infant, partner, Dysfunctional
relationship between parents/nurturing
figures, Situational crisis (specific to
family)

Post-Trauma Response
Related factors: Abuse, Assault,
Torture, Accidents, Incest, Rape

Self-Esteem Disturbance
Related factor: Abuse

Sleep Pattern Disturbance
Related factors: Anxiety, Emotional
state

Social Interaction, Impaired
Related factor: Concept disturbance

Violence, High Risk: Directed at others
Risk factor: History of physical/mental
abuse by others

■ CHRONIC ILLNESS: DEVELOPMENTAL PROBLEMS/NEEDS

Activity Intolerance
Related factors: Decreased strength and endurance, Weakness/fatigue, Imbalance between oxygen supply and demand, Pain (acute or chronic)

Activity Intolerance: High Risk
Risk factors: Limited mobility, Frail or debilitated states, Chronic illness, Pain

Adjustment, Impaired
Related factors: Incomplete grieving, Necessity for major life-style/behavior change, Pattern of dependence, Inadequate support systems

Anxiety
Related factors: Threat to or change in role functioning, Threat to or change in interaction patterns, Unmet needs

Body Image Disturbance
Related factors: Chronic illness, Chronic pain, Treatment side-effects

Caregiver Role Strain (Actual/High Risk)
Related factors/risk factors: Illness severity of the care receiver, Premature birth/congenital defect, Developmental delay or retardation of the care receiver, Marginal caregiver's coping patterns, Duration of caregiving required, Caregiver's competing role commitments, Complexity/amount of caregiving tasks, Lack of respite and recreation for caregiver

Family Processes, Altered
Related factors: Change in family roles, Illness/disability of family member, Unmet expectations for child, Lack of adequate support systems

Fear
Related factors: Powerlessness, Real threat to own well-being

Grieving, Dysfunctional
Related factors: Loss (actual or anticipated), Chronic illness

Growth and Development, Altered
Related factors: Serious illness, Prescribed dependence/limitations

Home Maintenance Management, Impaired
Related factors: Home environment obstacles, Inadequate support system, Insufficient family organization or planning, Insufficient finances, Lack of familiarity with community resources, Developmental disability

Hopelessness
Related factor: Failing or deteriorating physical condition

Knowledge Deficit (specify)
Related factors: Specific to patient, Specific to parent

Noncompliance
Related factors: Denial of illness, Negative consequence of treatment regimen, Perceived benefits of continued illness

Nutrition, Altered: Less Than Body Requirements
Related factor: Chronic illness

Pain, Chronic
Related factors: Specific to patient

Parenting, Altered
Related factors: Interruption in bonding process, Treatment-imposed separation, Lack of knowledge/skill necessary to address the child's special needs

Powerlessness
Related factor: Chronic illness

Role Performance, Altered
Related factors: Chronic illness, Chronic pain

Self-Care Deficit: Bathing/Hygiene, Dressing/Grooming, Feeding, Toileting (specify)
Related factors: Depression, Pain/discomfort, Intolerance to activity, Decreased strength and endurance

Self-Esteem Disturbance
Related factors: Chronic illness, Chronic pain

Social Interaction, Impaired
Related factors: Self-concept disturbance, Limited physical mobility

Spiritual Distress
Related factor: Test of spiritual beliefs

■ CLEFT LIP/CLEFT PALATE:
SURGICAL REPAIR

Airway Clearance, Ineffective
Related factor: Edema secondary to surgery

Body Image Disturbance
Related factor: Obvious congenital anomaly

Family Processes, Altered
Related factors: Hospitalization/change in environment, Illness/disability of family member, Separation of family members

Fear
Related factors: Environmental stressors/hospitalization, Separation from parent

Fluid Volume Deficit: High Risk
Risk factor: Deviation affecting access to or intake of fluids secondary to difficult handling of oral fluids

Infant Feeding Pattern, Ineffective
Related factors: Anatomical abnormalities, Oral hypersensitivity

Infection: High Risk
Risk factor: Trauma secondary to surgery

Injury: High Risk (Disruption of Surgical Site)
Risk factors: Limitations of maturational age, Tension on suture line secondary to crying

Nutrition, Altered: Less Than Body Requirements
Related factors: Difficulty in chewing, Difficulty in swallowing secondary to acute pain

Oral Mucous Membrane, Altered
Related factor: Surgery in oral cavity

Pain [Acute]
Related factor: Surgical repair of cleft lip/palate

Parenting, Altered
Related factors: Interruption in bonding process, Lack of knowledge/skill in special needs of child, Treatment-imposed separation

Self-Care Deficit: Feeding
Related factors: Age of child and need for adapted feeding

■ COAGULATION DISORDERS

Include but are not limited to hemophilia, von Willebrand's disease, idiopathic thrombocytopenic purpura.

Activity Intolerance: High Risk
Risk factors: Limited mobility, Pain, Fatigue

Coping, Ineffective Individual
Related factors: Chronic illness and limitations

Family Processes, Altered
Related factors: Illness/disability of family member, Environmental stressors/hospitalization

Fear
Related factors: Risks associated with diagnosis (uncontrollable bleeding, potential joint degeneration, risk of transfusion-acquired diseases)

Growth and Development, Altered
Related factors: Serious illness, Prescribed dependence/limitations

Injury: High Risk
Risk factor: Uncontrolled bleeding

Knowledge Deficit (specify)
Related factors: Lack of exposure to information about prevention of bleeding and injury and early recognition of bleeding, Cognitive limitations, Unreadiness to learn

Pain [Acute]
Related factor: Joint hemorrhage

Parenting, Altered
Related factors: Lack of knowledge/skill in care of special child, Treatment-imposed separation

Powerlessness
Related factor: Chronic illness

Role Performance, Altered
Related factor: Chronic illness

Self-Esteem Disturbance
Related factor: Chronic illness

■ CONGENITAL MALFORMATIONS OF THE CENTRAL NERVOUS SYSTEM: SURGICAL REPAIR

Include but are not limited to spina bifida, meningocele, myelomeningocele, hydrocephalus.

Caregiver Role Strain (Actual/High Risk)
Related factors/risk factors: Illness severity of the care receiver, Congenital defect, Developmental delay of care receiver, Caregiver's competing role commitments, Lack of respite and recreation for caregiver

Diversional Activity Deficit
Related factors: Forced inactivity, Prolonged bed rest, Long-term hospitalization

Family Processes, Altered
Related factors: Hospitalization/change in environment, Illness/disability of family member, Separation of family members

Fear (parental)
Related factor: Real threat to child

Infection: High Risk
Risk factor: Broken skin secondary to surgery

Injury: High Risk
Risk factor: Increased intracranial pressure/seizures secondary to shunt malfunction in hydrocephalus

Knowledge Deficit (Parental)
Related factor: Limited exposure to information (home care)

Mobility, Impaired Physical
Related factor: Neuromuscular impairment secondary to spinal cord involvement

Pain [Acute]
Related factor: Surgery

Parenting, Altered
Related factors: Interruption in bonding process, Lack of knowledge/skill in needs of special child, Treatment-imposed separation

Self-Care Deficit: Bathing/Hygiene, Dressing/Grooming, Feeding, Toileting (specify)
Related factor: Neuromuscular impairment

Sensory/Perceptual Alterations: Kinesthetic, Tactile
Related factor: Sensory deficits secondary to spinal cord involvement

Skin Integrity, Impaired: High Risk
Risk factors: Immobility, Incontinence of stool/urine

■ FAILURE TO THRIVE

Activity Intolerance
Related factors: Weakness/fatigue

Coping, Ineffective Family: Disabling
Related factors: Chronically unresolved feelings, Highly ambivalent family relationships

Family Processes, Altered
Related factors: Unmet expectations for child, Hospitalization/change in environment

Fluid Volume Deficit
Related factors: Inadequate fluid intake secondary to disinterest in eating/drinking, Abnormal fluid loss (loose stools)

Infant Feeding Pattern, Ineffective
Related factor: Prolonged NPO

Infection: High Risk
Risk factor: Malnutrition

Nutrition, Altered: Less Than Body Requirements
Related factors: Food intolerance, Malabsorption, Loss of appetite, Parental neglect

Parenting, Altered
Related factors: Lack of or inappropriate response of child to parent, Lack of knowledge/skill, Absent or ineffective role model, Interruption in bonding process

Skin Integrity, Impaired: High Risk
Risk factor: Altered nutritional status

Social Interaction, Impaired
Related factors: Developmental disability, Limited physical mobility

■ **GASTROENTERITIS**

Diarrhea
Related factors: Food intolerance, Stress, Dietary changes, Increased intestinal motility

Family Processes, Altered
Related factors: Hospitalization/change in environment, Separation of family members

Fear
Related factors: Environmental stressors/hospitalization, Real or imagined threat to own well-being

Fluid Volume Deficit
Related factors: Abnormal fluid loss (diarrhea) secondary to infection, Food intolerance, Inflammatory disease, Malabsorption

Nutrition, Altered: Less Than Body Requirements
Related factors: Loss of appetite, Nausea/vomiting

Oral Mucous Membrane, Altered
Related factor: Dehydration

Pain [Acute]
Related factor: Muscle cramps (abdominal)

Sensory/Perceptual Alterations: Visual, Auditory, Kinesthetic, Tactile (specify)
Related factor: Electrolyte imbalance

Skin Integrity, Impaired: High Risk
Risk factors: Incontinence of stool, Diarrhea

■ **GASTROINTESTINAL OBSTRUCTION: SURGICAL REPAIR**

Includes but is not limited to gastroschisis, omphalocele, intestinal atresia, meconium ileus, imperforate anus, Hirschsprung's disease, pyloric stenosis, intussusception, inguinal hernia, and hydrocele.

Activity Intolerance
Related factors: Acute pain, Decreased strength and endurance

Breathing Pattern, Ineffective
Related factor: Acute pain

Family Processes, Altered
Related factors: Illness/disability of family member, Hospitalization/change in environment, Separation of family members

Fear
Related factors: Environmental stressors/hospitalization, Real threat to well-being

Fluid Volume Deficit
Related factors: Abnormal blood loss, Abnormal fluid loss

Nutrition, Altered: Less Than Body Requirements
Related factors: Loss of appetite, Nausea/vomiting

Pain [Acute]
Related factor: Surgery

Parenting, Altered
Related factors: Lack of knowledge/skill in special needs of child

Skin Integrity, Impaired: High Risk
Risk factors: Altered nutritional status, Surgical wound

■ INFECTION OF CENTRAL
  NERVOUS SYSTEM

Includes but is not limited to meningitis, encephalitis, rabies, Reye's syndrome, Guillain-Barré syndrome.

**Caregiver Role Strain
(Actual/High Risk)**
Related factors/risk factors: Illness severity of the care receiver, Duration of caregiving required, Caregiver's competing role commitments

Communication, Impaired: Verbal
Related factor: Inability to speak secondary to coma

Family Processes, Altered
Related factors: Illness of child, Separation of family members

Fear (Parental)
Related factor: Real threat to child

Fluid Volume Deficit
Related factors: Inadequate fluid intake secondary to nausea, Abnormal fluid loss secondary to vomiting

Grieving, Anticipatory (Parental)
Related factor: Anticipated loss of child

Injury: High Risk
Risk factor: Seizure activity

Mobility, Physical, Impaired
Related factors: Neuromuscular impairment, Coma

Pain [Acute]
Related factors: Nausea/vomiting, Headache, Paresthesia

**Self-Care Deficit: Bathing/Hygiene,
Dressing/Grooming, Feeding,
Toileting (specify)**
Related factors: Neuromuscular impairment, Coma

**Sensory/Perceptual Alterations: Visual,
Auditory, Kinesthetic, Gustatory,
Tactile, Olfactory (specify)**
Related factor: Sensory deficits secondary to coma

■ INGESTION/ACCIDENTAL POISONING

Breathing Pattern, Ineffective
Related factor: Depression of respiratory center secondary to ___ (specify drug)

Family Processes, Altered
Related factors: Hospitalization/change in environment, Illness/disability of family member, Separation of family members, Parental guilt

Fluid Volume Excess
Related factor: Decreased urine output secondary to renal dysfunction

Gas Exchange, Impaired
Related factor: Anemia secondary to lead poisoning

**Home Maintenance Management,
Impaired**
Related factors: Lack of knowledge about prevention of accidental poisoning, Insufficient family organization or planning

Injury: High Risk
Risk factor: Seizures secondary to lead poisoning, aspirin toxicity

**Sensory/Perceptual Alterations: Visual,
Auditory, Kinesthetic, Gustatory,
Tactile, Olfactory (specify)**
Related factors: Decreased consciousness, Encephalopathy

■ OBESE CHILD

Body Image Disturbance
Related factor: Eating disorder (obesity)

Coping, Ineffective Family: Disabling
Related factors: Arbitrary disregard for child's needs, Conflicting coping styles, Highly ambivalent relationships

Health Maintenance, Altered
Related factors: Cultural beliefs, Lack of social supports, Lack of ability to make deliberate and thoughtful judgments secondary to maturational age

Nutrition, Altered: More Than Body Requirements
Related factors: Psychologic impairment, Sedentary life-style, Lack of basic nutritional knowledge, Ethnic/cultural norms

Self-Esteem Disturbance
Related factor: Obesity

Social Interaction, Impaired
Related factor: Self-concept disturbance

Social Isolation
Related factor: Obesity

■ OSTEOMYELITIS

Activity Intolerance
Related factor: Acute pain

Diversional Activity Deficit
Related factors: Long-term hospitalization, Forced inactivity

Family Processes, Altered
Related factors: Illness/disability of family member, Hospitalization/change in environment, Separation of family members

Mobility, Impaired Physical
Related factors: Pain/discomfort, Medically prescribed limitations, Musculoskeletal impairment

Nutrition, Altered: Less Than Body Requirements
Related factor: High metabolic state

Pain [Acute]
Related factor: Inflammation

Self-Care Deficit: Bathing/Hygiene, Dressing/Grooming, Feeding, Toileting (specify)
Related factors: Pain/discomfort, Decreased strength and endurance, Neuromuscular impairment

Social Interaction, Impaired
Related factor: Limited physical mobility

■ PREGNANCY IN ADOLESCENCE

Includes pregnancy, antepartum and postpartum periods, and parenting

Body Image Disturbance
Related factor: Pregnancy

Coping, Ineffective Individual
Related factors: Adolescent pregnancy, Adolescent parenthood

Family Processes, Altered
Related factors: Lack of adequate support systems, Change in family roles

Fear
Related factors: Threat to own well-being, Powerlessness

Health Maintenance, Altered
Related factors: Lack of social supports, Lack of material resources, Cultural beliefs, Lack of ability to make deliberate and thoughtful judgments secondary to maturational age

Home Maintenance Management, Impaired
Related factors: Inadequate support system, Insufficient family organization or planning, Insufficient finances, Lack of familiarity with community resources

Knowledge Deficit (specify)
Related factors: Limited exposure to information (birth control, parenting), Limited practice of skills, Information misinterpretation

Nutrition, Altered: Less Than Body Requirements
Related factors: High metabolic needs, Lack of basic nutritional knowledge, Limited access to food, Nausea/vomiting

Nutrition, Altered: More Than Body Requirements
Related factors: Ethnic/cultural norms, Lack of basic nutritional knowledge

Parenting, Altered
Related factors: Lack of knowledge/
skill, Lack of support for nurturing
figure, Unrealistic expectations of self/
infant/partner, Situational crisis

Role Performance, Altered
Related factors: Assumption of new
role, Unmet expectations for pregnancy,
Unmet expectations for childbirth

Social Interaction, Impaired
Related factors: Sociocultural conflict,
Self-concept disturbance

Social Isolation
Related factors: Alteration in physical
appearance, Life-style changes

Violence, High Risk: Directed at Child
Risk factors: Rage reaction, History of
physical/mental abuse by others,
Substance abuse

See also *Antepartum and Postpartum
Conditions,* pp. 293–299

■ RESPIRATORY DISORDER, CHRONIC

Includes but is not limited to asthma,
bronchopulmonary dysplasia, cystic fibrosis.

Activity Intolerance
Related factors: Imbalance between
oxygen supply and demand, Anxiety,
Weakness/fatigue, Decreased strength
and endurance

Adjustment, Impaired
Related factors: Necessity for major life-
style/behavior changes, Pattern of
dependence

Airway Clearance, Ineffective
Related factors: Tracheobronchial
secretions, Spasms of the bronchi and
bronchioles

Body Image Disturbance
Related factor: Chronic illness

Breathing Pattern, Ineffective
Related factors: Anxiety, Pulmonary
infection, Decreased energy/fatigue

**Caregiver Role Strain
(Actual/High Risk)**
Related factors/risk factors: Illness
severity of the care receiver, Caregiver's
competing role commitments, Complex-
ity/amount of caregiving tasks, Duration
of the caregiving required, Lack of
respite and recreation for caregiver

Coping, Ineffective Individual
Related factor: Stressors of chronic
illness

Fluid Volume Deficit: High Risk
Risk factors: Inadequate fluid intake
secondary to difficulty in breathing,
Abnormal fluid loss secondary to
increased insensible water loss from
rapid respirations

Gas Exchange, Impaired
Related factor: Decreased functional
lung tissue secondary to fibrotic,
nonventilated areas of lung parenchyma
in bronchopulmonary dysplasia

Infection: High Risk
Risk factors: Malnutrition, Stasis of
respiratory secretions

Knowledge Deficit (specify)
Related factors: Limited exposure to
information, Limited practice of skill

**Nutrition, Altered: Less Than Body
Requirements**
Related factors: Loss of appetite with
chronic illness, High metabolic needs
secondary to pulmonary infection,
Malabsorption of nutrients secondary to
cystic fibrosis

Parenting, Altered
Related factors: Lack of knowledge/skill
in care of special child, Treatment-
imposed separation

Powerlessness
Related factor: Chronic illness

Role Performance, Altered
Related factor: Chronic illness

Self-Care Deficit: Bathing/Hygiene, Dressing/Grooming, Feeding, Toileting (specify)
Related factors: Intolerance to activity, Developmental disability

Self-Esteem Disturbance
Related factor: Chronic illness

Social Interaction, Impaired
Related factors: Developmental disability, Self-concept disturbance

Social Isolation
Related factors: Medical condition, Alteration in physical appearance, Lifestyle changes

■ **RESPIRATORY INFECTION, ACUTE**

Includes but is not limited to tonsillitis, pharyngitis, croup, laryngotracheobronchitis, epiglottitis, bronchitis, pneumonia.

Activity Intolerance
Related factors: Imbalance between oxygen supply/demand, Weakness/fatigue

Airway Clearance, Ineffective
Related factors: Edema, Tracheobronchial secretions

Diversional Activity Deficit
Related factor: Time spent in croupette

Family Processes, Altered
Related factors: Illness/disability of family member, Hospitalization/change in environment, Separation of family members

Fear
Related factors: Real threat to well-being, Environmental stressors/hospitalization, Separation from parent

Fluid Volume Deficit: High Risk
Risk factors: Inadequate fluid intake secondary to difficulty in breathing, Abnormal fluid loss secondary to increased insensible water loss from rapid respirations

Gas Exchange, Impaired
Related factor: Decreased functional lung tissue secondary to pneumonia

Nutrition, Altered: Less Than Body Requirements
Related factors: Loss of appetite, High metabolic needs

Pain [Acute]
Related factors: Sore throat, Pain with inspiration

Sensory/Perceptual Alterations: Visual, Auditory, Kinesthetic, Tactile (specify)
Related factor: Sensory deficit secondary to time spent in croupette

Skin Integrity, Impaired: High Risk
Risk factors: Altered nutritional status, Hyperthermia, Damp therapeutic environment

■ **SEIZURE DISORDERS**

Adjustment, Impaired
Related factors: Assault to self-esteem, Incomplete grieving

Anxiety
Related factors: Threat to role functioning, Change in role functioning

Family Processes, Altered
Related factors: Hospitalization/change in environment, Illness/disability of family member, Separation of family members

Fear
Related factor: Real threat to own well-being

Injury: High Risk
Risk factor: Seizure activity

Knowledge Deficit (specify)
Related factors: Specific to patient, Specific to parent

Noncompliance
Related factors: Denial of illness, Negative perception of treatment regimen, Perceived benefits of continued illness

Powerlessness
Related factor: Chronic illness

Self-Esteem Disturbance
Related factor: Chronic illness

Social Interaction, Impaired
Related factor: Self-concept disturbance

■ SEPSIS

Breathing Pattern, Ineffective
Related factors: Decreased energy/fatigue

Constipation
Related factor: Decreased fluid intake

Diarrhea
Related factor: Increased intestinal motility

Family Processes, Altered
Related factors: Illness/disability of family member, Separation of family members

Fluid Volume Deficit: High Risk
Risk factors: Decreased fluid intake, Fever

Injury: High Risk
Risk factor: Seizure activity secondary to high fever

Nutrition, Altered: Less Than Body Requirements
Related factors: Inadequate sucking reflex in infant, Vomiting, Food intolerance, High metabolic state, Lethargy

Skin Integrity, Impaired: High Risk
Risk factors: Decreased peripheral perfusion, Hyperthermia

Sleep Pattern Disturbance
Related factor: Sleep deprivation secondary to frequent therapeutic interventions

■ SICKLE CELL CRISIS

Activity Intolerance
Related factor: Imbalance between oxygen supply/demand

Family Processes, Altered
Related factors: Illness of family member, Hospitalization/change in environment

Fear
Related factors: Environmental stressors/hospitalization, Real threat to well-being of child

Fluid Volume Deficit
Related factor: Increased need for fluid volume in blood to prevent sickling and thrombosis

Gas Exchange, Impaired
Related factor: Decreased pulmonary blood supply secondary to anemia

Infection: High Risk
Risk factor: Chronic illness

Knowledge Deficit (specify)
Related factors: Limited exposure to information about prevention of sickle cell crisis by minimizing oxygen needs of body, Cognitive limitations, Unreadiness to learn

Pain [Acute]
Related factor: Sickle cell crisis

Tissue Perfusion, Altered: Peripheral
Related factors: Imbalance between oxygen supply/demand secondary to anemia, Thrombosis secondary to clumping of red blood cells in sickle cell crisis

■ TONSILLECTOMY

Airway Clearance, Ineffective
Related factors: Trauma, Edema, Pain, Tracheobronchial secretions

Family Processes, Altered
Related factors: Hospitalization/change in environment, Separation of family members

Fear
Related factors: Environmental stressors/hospitalization, Surgical procedure

Nutrition, Altered: Less Than Body Requirements
Related factor: Loss of appetite

Oral Mucous Membrane, Altered
Related factor: Surgery in oral cavity

Pain [Acute]
Related factor: Surgery

▪ Bibliography

Acute Pain Management Guideline Panel. (Feb. 1992). *Acute Pain Management: Operative or Medical Procedures and Trauma. Clinical Practice Guideline.* AHCPR Pub. No. 92-0032. Rockville, MD: Agency for Health Care Policy and Research, Public Health Service, U.S. Department of Health and Human Services.

Anderson, L., and Price, C. (1986). Nursing care of patients with pulmonary insufficiency. *Critical Care Nursing Currents.* Vol. 4, No. 4, 19–34.

Auerbach, K. G. (1990). Assisting the employed breastfeeding mother. *Journal of Nurse-Midwifery,* Vol. 35, No. 1, 26–34.

Ballard, P. (1983). Breast-feeding for the working mother. *Issues in Comprehensive Pediatric Nursing,* Vol. 6, 249–259.

Bower, K. (1991). Introduction to case management: A three-hour workshop. El Camino Hospital, Mountain View, CA.

Bowers, B. (1987). Intergenerational caregiving: Adult caregivers and their aging parents. *Advances in Nursing Science,* Vol. 9, No. 2, 20–31.

Carnevali, Doris. (1984). Nursing diagnosis: An evolutionary view. *Topics in Clinical Nursing.* Vol. 5, No. 4, 10–20.

Carpenito, Lynda J. (1991). *Nursing Diagnosis: Application to Clinical Practice.* Philadelphia, PA: J. P. Lippincott.

Carroll, J., Schaffer, C. B., Spensley, J., and Abramowitz, S. (1981). Family antecedents of adult self-mutilators. *International Journal of Family Psychiatry,* Vol. 2, Nos. 1 & 2, 147–161.

Chilman, C., Nunnally, E., and Cox, F. (1988). *Chronic Illness and Disability.* Beverly Hills, CA: Sage Publications. 30–31.

Conn, L. M., and Lion, J. R. (1983). Self-mutilation: A review. *Psychiatric Medicine,* Vol. 1, No. 1, 21–33.

Cook, J. S., and Fontaine, K. L. (1987). Violence against others—Rape. *Essentials of Mental Health Nursing.* Menlo Park, CA: Addison-Wesley. 522–530.

Cox, C. (1985). The health self-determinism index. *Nursing Research,* Vol. 34, No. 3, 177–183.

Doughty, D. (Ed.). (1991). *Urinary and Fecal Incontinence: Nursing Management.* St. Louis, MO: Mosby-Yearbook.

El Camino Hospital Care Delivery Task Force. (1991). Objectives for new care delivery system. El Camino Hospital, Mountain View, CA.

El Camino Hospital Clinical Practice Council. (1992). *Management of the Adult Patient Being Weaned.* El Camino Hospital, Mountain View, CA.

Favazza, A. R. (1989). Why patients mutilate themselves. *Hospital and Community Psychiatry,* Vol. 40, No. 2, 137–145.

Figueroa, M. (1988). A dynamic taxonomy of self-destructive behavior. *Psychotherapy,* Vol. 25, No. 2, 280–287.

Fitzpatrick, Joyce J., et al. (1989). Translating nursing diagnosis into ICD code. *American Journal of Nursing.* Vol. 89, No. 4, 483–495.

Forte, A., Mayberry, L. J., and Ferketich, S. (1987). Breast milk collection and storage practices among mothers of hospitalized neonates. *Journal of Perinatology,* Vol. 7, No. 1, 35–39.

Gray, M. (1992). *Genitourinary Disorders.* St. Louis, MO: Mosby-Yearbook.

Gyulay, Jo-Eileen. (1989). Grief responses. *Issues in Comprehensive Pediatric Nursing,* Vol. 12, No. 1, 1–31.

Halpern, J. S., (1989). Clinical notebook: Lower extremity peripheral nerve assessment. *Journal of Emergency Nursing,* Vol. 15, No. 4, 333–337.

Hawkins-Walsh, E. (1988). Breastfeeding the premature infant. *Pediatric Nursing Forum,* Vol. 3, No. 4, 3–13.

Henneman, E. A. (1991). The art and science of weaning from mechanical ventilation. *AACN Focus on Critical Care,* Vol. 18, No. 6, 490–501.

Hilt, N. E., and Cogburn, S. B. (1980). *Manual of Orthopaedics.* St. Louis, MO: C. V. Mosby, 487–537.

Hurley, Mary (Ed.). (1986). *Classification of Nursing Diagnoses: Proceedings of the Sixth Conference, North American Nursing Diagnosis Association.* St. Louis, MO: C. V. Mosby.

International Association of Enterostomal Therapy. (1987). *Standards of Care, Dermal Wounds: Pressure Sores.* Irvine, CA.

Jenny, J., and Logan, J. (1991). Analyzing expert nursing practice to develop a new nursing diagnosis: Dysfunctional ventilatory weaning response. In R. M. Carroll-Johnson. (Ed.) *Classification of Nursing Diagnoses: Proceedings of the Ninth Conference.* Philadelphia, PA: J. P. Lippincott, 133–140.

Johnson, Sharon E. (1988). Alteration in temperature regulation: Hypothermia. *Classifications of Nursing Diagnoses: Proceedings of the Eighth Conference, North American Nursing Diagnosis Association.* St. Louis, MO: C. V. Mosby. 378–380.

Jones, R., et al. (Nov. 1974). *Patient Classification for Long-Term Care: User's Manual.* HEW Publ. No. HRA-74-3107.

Knebel, A. F. (1991). Weaning from mechanical ventilation: Current controversies. *Heart & Lung,* Vol. 20, No. 4, 321–333.

Kriteck, Phyllis. (1986). Diagnostics: The struggle to classify our diagnoses. *American Journal of Nursing,* Vol. 86, No. 6, 722–723.

Laffrey, S. C., and Crabtree, M. K. (1988). Health and health behavior of persons with chronic cardiovascular disease. *International Journal of Nursing Studies,* Vol. 25, No. 1, 41–52.

Logan, J., and Jenny, J. (1991) Interventions for the nursing diagnosis. Dysfunctional ventilatory weaning response: A qualitative study. In R. M. Carroll-Johnson. (Ed.) *Classification of Nursing Diagnoses: Proceedings of the Ninth Conference,* Philadelphia, PA: J. P. Lippincott, 141–147.

Loomis, M., et al. (1986). *Classification of Individual Human Responses of Concern for Psychiatric/Mental Health Nursing Practice.* Unpublished draft. American Nurses' Association Subcommittee.

Lubkin, I. M. (1986). Compliance. In *Chronic Illness: Impact and Interventions.* Boston, MA: Jones and Bartlett, 126–149.

McCaffrey, M. (1979). *Nursing Management of the Patient with Pain.* Second Edition. Philadelphia, PA: J. P. Lippincott.

McLane, A. (Ed.). (1987). *Classification of Nursing Diagnoses: Proceedings of the Seventh Conference, North American Nursing Diagnosis Association.* St. Louis, MO: C. V. Mosby.

Marculescu, Gail. (1986). *The Nursing Diagnosis Disturbance in Self-Concept, Related to a Change in Body Image in Post-Surgical Patients: A Descriptive Study.* Unpublished Master's Thesis. San Jose State University.

Marini, J. J. (1986). The physiologic determinants of ventilator dependency. *Respiratory Care,* Vol. 31, 271–282.

Matz, R. (1986). Hypothermia: Measures and countermeasures. *Hospital Practice,* Vol. 21, No. 1A, 45–71.

Mirotznik, J., and Ruskin, A. P. (1985). Inter-institutional relocation and its effects on psychosocial status. *The Gerontologist,* Vol. 25, No. 3, 265–270.

Mott, S., James, S., and Sperhac, A. (1990). *Nursing Care of Children and Families.* Menlo Park, CA: Addison-Wesley.

Neifert, M., and Seacat, J. (1986). Medical management of successful breastfeeding. *Pediatric Clinics of North America,* Vol. 33, No. 4, 743–762.

North American Nursing Diagnosis Association. (1986). Seventh Conference on Classification of Nursing Diagnoses. *Syllabus of Conference Proceedings.* NANDA, St. Louis, MO.

North American Nursing Diagnosis Association. (1988). Eighth Conference on Classification of Nursing Diagnoses. *Syllabus of Conference Proceedings.* NANDA, St. Louis.

North American Nursing Diagnosis Association. (1988). *Nursing Diagnosis Newsletter,*Vol. 31, No. 1.

North American Nursing Diagnosis Association. (1989). *Taxonomy I, Revised.* NANDA, St. Louis, MO.

Norton, L. C., and Neureuter, A. (1989). Weaning the long-term ventilator dependent patient: Common problems and management. *Critical Care Nurse,* Vol. 9, No. 1, 42–51.

Orzeck, Susan, and Ouslander, Joseph. (1987). Urinary incontinence: An overview of causes and treatment. *Journal of Enterostomal Therapy,* Vol. 14, No. 1, 20–27.

Panel for the Prediction and Prevention of Pressure Ulcers in Adults. (May 1992). *Pressure Ulcers in Adults: Prediction and Prevention. Clinical Practice Guideline Number 3.* AHCPR Pub. No. 92-0047. Rockville, MD: Agency for Health Care Policy and Research, Public Health Service, U.S. Department of Health and Human Services.

Pattison, E. M., and Kahan, J. (1983). The deliberate self-harm syndrome. *American Journal of Psychiatry,* Vol. 140, No. 7, 867–872.

Rantz, K. E. (1987). Reducing death from translocation syndrome. *American Journal of Nursing,* Vol. 87, 1351–1352.

Reuler, J. (1978). Hypothermia: Pathophysiology, clinical settings, and management. *Annals of Internal Medicine,* Vol. 89, 519–527.

Rhynsburger, J. (1989). How to fight MG fatigue. *American Journal of Nursing,* Vol. 89, 337–340.

Schactman, M. (1987). Transfer stress in patients after myocardial infarction. *Focus on Critical Care,* Vol. 14, No. 2, 34–37.

Schainen, J. S. (1991). Environments for nursing care of the older client. In W. C. Chenitz, J. T. Stone, and S. A. Salisbury, *Clinical Gerontological Nursing.* Philadelphia, PA: W. B. Saunders.

Seifert, Patricia, and Grandsky, Rosemary. (1990). Nursing diagnoses: Their use in developing care plans. *AORN Journal,* Vol. 51, No. 4, 1008–1021.

Shaker, C. (1990). Nipple feeding premature infants: A different perspective. *Neonatal Network,* Vol. 8, No. 5, 9–17.

Sheppard, Kathleen. (1987). Alterations in protective mechanisms. *Classification of Nursing Diagnoses: Proceedings of the Seventh Conference, North American Nursing Diagnosis Association.* St. Louis, MO: C. V. Mosby. 239–246.

Sheppard, Kathleen. (1988). Validation of the nursing diagnosis "alterations in protective mechanisms." *Classification of Nursing Diagnoses: Proceedings of the Eighth Conference, North American Nursing Diagnosis Association.* St. Louis, MO: C. V. Mosby. 281–283.

Smith, Linda. (1987). Sexual assault: The nurse's role. *AD Nurse,* Vol. 2, No. 2, 24–28.

Stevens, S. A., and Becker, K. L. (Sept. 1988). A simple, step-by-step approach to neurologic assessment, part 1. *Nursing,* 53–61.

Stine, M. J. (1990). Breastfeeding the premature newborn: A protocol without bottles. *Journal of Human Lactation,* Vol. 6, No. 4, 167–170.

Taylor, Cynthia, and Cress, Sheila. (1992). *The Indispensable Care Plan Guide— Nursing Diagnosis Cards.* Springhouse, PA: Springhouse Corporation.

Thompson, J., et al. (1989). *Mosby's Manual of Clinical Nursing.* Second Edition. St. Louis, MO: C. V. Mosby.

Urinary Incontinence Guideline Panel. (March 1992). *Urinary Incontinence in Adults: Clinical Practice Guideline.* AHCPR Pub. No 92-0038. Rockville, MD: Agency for Health Care Policy and Research, Public Health Service, U.S. Department of Health and Human Services.

Voith, Anne-Marie. (1986). A conceptual framework for nursing diagnoses: Alterations in urinary elimination. *Rehabilitation Nursing,* Vol. 11, No. 1, 18–20.

Walsh, B. W., and Rosen, P. M. (1988). *Self-Mutilation: Theory, Research, and Treatment.* New York, NY: The Guilford Press.

Yang, K. L., and Tobin, M. J. (1991). A prospective study of indexes predicting the outcome of trials of weaning from mechanical ventilation. *New England Journal of Medicine,* Vol. 324, No. 21, 1445–1451.

Youll, James W. (1989). The bridge beyond: Strengthening nursing practice in attitudes towards death, dying, and the terminally ill, and helping the spouses of critically ill patients. *Intensive Care Nursing,* Vol. 5, No. 2, 88–94.

■ Appendix

NANDA's Taxonomy I Revised

Human Response Pattern: Choosing
(A human response pattern involving the selection of alternatives)

*Y00 Family Coping, Impaired
  Y00.0 Compromised
  Y00.1 Disabled
Y01 [Health-Seeking Behaviors]
  Y01.0–9 Health Seeking Behaviors
    (Specify)
*Y02 Individual Coping, Impaired
  Y02.0 Adjustment, Impaired
  Y02.1 Conflict: Decisional
  Y02.2 Coping: Defensive
  *Y02.3 Denial, Impaired
  Y02.4 Noncompliance

Human Response Pattern: Communicating
(A human response pattern involving the sending of messages)

Y10 [Communication, Impaired]
  Y10.0 Verbal

Human Response Pattern: Exchanging
(A human response pattern involving mutual giving and receiving)

Y20 [Bowel Elimination, Altered]
  Y20.0 Bowel Incontinence
  Y20.1 Constipation: Colonic
  Y20.2 Constipation: Perceived
  Y20.3 Diarrhea
*Y21 Cardiac Output, Altered
Y22 [Fluid Volume, Altered]
  Y22.0 Deficit
  Y22.1 Deficit: Risk
  Y22.2 Excess
*Y23 Injury: Risk
  *Y23.0 Aspiration
  *Y23.1 Disuse Syndrome
  *Y23.2 Poisoning
  *Y23.3 Suffocation
  *Y23.4 Trauma

Y24 [Nutrition, Altered]
  Y24.0 Less than Body Requirement
  Y24.1 More than Body
    Requirement
  Y24.2 More than Body
    Requirement: Risk
Y25 [Physical Regulation, Altered]
  Y25.0 Dysreflexia
  Y25.1 Hyperthermia
  Y25.2 Hypothermia
  *Y25.3 Infection: Risk
  *Y25.4 Thermoregulation, Impaired
Y26 [Respiration, Altered]
  *Y26.0 Airway Clearance, Impaired
  *Y26.1 Breathing Pattern, Impaired
  Y26.2 Gas Exchange, Impaired
Y27 Tissue Integrity, Altered
  *Y27.0 Oral Mucous Membrane,
    Impaired
  Y27.1 Skin Integrity, Impaired
  Y27.2 Skin Integrity, Impaired: Risk
Y28 [Tissue Perfusion, Altered]
  Y28.0 Cardiopulmonary
  Y28.1 Cerebral
  Y28.2 Gastrointestinal
  Y28.3 Peripheral
  Y28.4 Renal
Y29 Urinary Elmination, Altered
  Y29.0 Incontinence: Functional
  Y29.1 Incontinence: Reflex
  Y29.2 Incontinence: Stress
  Y29.3 Incontinence: Urge
  Y29.4 Incontinence: Total
  *Y29.5 Retention

Human Response Pattern: Feeling
(A human response pattern involving the subjective awareness of information)

Y30 Anxiety
Y31 [Comfort, Altered]
  Y31.0 Pain [Acute]
  Y31.1 Pain Chronic
Y32 Fear

Y33 [Grieving]
Y33.0 Anticipatory
Y33.1 Dysfunctional
Y34 Post-Trauma Response
Y34.0 Rape Trauma Syndrome
Y34.1 Rape Trauma Syndrome: Compound Reaction
Y34.2 Rape Trauma Syndrome: Silent Reaction
*Y35 Violence: Risk

Human Response Pattern: Knowing
(A human response pattern involving the meaning associated with information)

Y40 [Knowledge Deficit]
Y40.0–9 Knowledge Deficit (Specify)
Y41 Thought Processes, Altered

Human Response Pattern: Moving
(A human response pattern involving activity)

Y50 [Activity, Altered]
Y50.0 Activity Intolerance
Y50.1 Activity Intolerance: Risk
Y50.2 Diversional Activity Deficit
Y50.3 Fatigue
Y50.4 Physical Mobility, Impaired
Y50.5 Sleep Pattern Disturbance
*Y51 Bathing/Hygiene Deficit
*Y52 Dressing/Grooming Deficit
*Y53 Feeding Deficit
*Y53.0 Breast-feeding, Impaired
Y53.1 Swallowing, Impaired
Y54 Growth and Development, Altered
Y55 Health Maintenance, Altered
Y56 Home Maintenance Management, Impaired
*Y57 Toileting Deficit

Human Response Pattern: Perceiving
(A human response pattern involving the reception of information)

Y60 [Meaningfulness, Altered]
Y60.0 Hopelessness
Y60.1 Powerlessness
Y61 [Self-Concept, Altered]
Y61.0 Body Image Disturbance
Y61.1 Personal Identity Disturbance
Y61.2 Self-Esteem Disturbance: Chronic Low
Y61.3 Self-Esteem Disturbance: Situational
*Y62 [Sensory Perception, Altered]
Y62.0 Auditory
Y62.1 Gustatory
Y62.2 Kinesthetic
Y62.3 Olfactory
Y62.4 Tactile
Y62.5 Visual
Y62.6 Unilateral Neglect

Human Response Pattern: Relating
(A human response pattern involving establishment of bonds)

Y70 Family Processes, Altered
Y71 Role Performance, Altered
Y71.0 Parental Role Conflict
Y71.1 Parenting, Altered
Y71.2 Parenting, Altered: Risk
Y71.3 Sexual Dysfunction
Y72 Sexuality Patterns, Altered
Y73 [Socialization, Altered]
Y73.0 Social Interaction, Impaired
Y73.1 Social Isolation

Human Response Pattern: Valuing
(A human response pattern involving the assigning of relative worth)

Y80 [Spiritual State, Altered]
Y80.0 Spiritual Distress

Note:

Items in brackets are not diagnoses accepted by NANDA.
Items with an asterisk (*) are changes in terminology from NANDA diagnostic labels.

Reference:

NANDA Board of Directors, Taxonomy Committee and ANA Liaison, January 28, 1989.

■ Index

Index